GW00597175

Angels at our Table

2nd Edition

Compiled by

ANN BREEN

ORIGINAL WRITING

ISBNs
PARENT: 978-1-906018-22-1
EPUB: 978-1-78237-140-3
MOBI: 978-1-78237-141-0
PDF: 978-1-78237-142-7

A CIP catalogue for this book is available from the
National Library.

Published by Original Writing Ltd., Dublin, 2007.

Printed in Great Britain by MPG BOOKS GROUP, Bodmin and Kings Lynn

For Paschal and Mark

with thanks for all the loving
support over the years

Contents

Foreword

Dear Ann,

It is a pleasure to write a few words as Patron about the Williams Syndrome Association of Ireland.

I remember, at our first meeting, your fears of the new-born organisation not taking off, for reasons of distance among other things and it is wonderful that you have managed to overcome these obstacles and form an efficient and effective group, spread out as it needs must be. Sharing information about WS with those affected by it is the most important role you face and your courage and perseverance have enabled you to win through and help others who were finding it hard to cope.

I send congratulations to you for devoting so much of your time in such a valuable and helpful way and I wish you well with the "Book of Stories." I am sure it will help many WS families in the future.

Desmond Guinness
Leixlip Castle
Leixlip
Co. Kildare

Introduction

MY FIRST "IRISH" CONTACT with Williams Syndrome came by way of a May 30 1986 letter from Ann Breen asking for more information about her newly diagnosed Williams Syndrome daughter, Karen. She finished her letter saying, "maybe you will be able to give me some hope for Karen's future." Ann was doubly perplexed because she was told there were only three cases, including Karen, in all of Ireland. I sent her information on June 12, 1986 and told her I would be in London and could meet them (Kathleen Giles and her affected son, Keith, also accompanied them) at the Gresham Hotel lobby at 10am to examine the two children and answer their questions about Williams Syndrome. We had a great 2–3 hour meeting while I enjoyed observing Karen and Keith. Among the many things we discussed was the fact that Williams Syndrome was not a rare condition (estimated prevalence 1 in 15,000) and that there should be between 30 and 50 cases in Ireland at the minimum. I suggested they talk with paediatric cardiologists and endocrinologists in Ireland to identify more cases with the intent of starting a parent support group for Ireland's Williams Syndrome children.

That seemed like a "good" idea to them and we parted with renewed enthusiasm and a plan.

On October 24, 1986 I received a follow-up letter from Kathleen Giles. She and Ann Breen had already met with Dr Desmond Duff (October 20, 1986), an Irish paediatric cardiologist who said he knew of 6 cases of Williams Syndrome and that he would write to the parents of those children to tell them about the developing Williams Syndrome Association of Ireland (WSAI). He also kindly offered to talk to other cardiologists about trying to identify additional cases. Ann's daughter's paediatrician, Dr Kevin Connolly, enthusiastically offered to contact other Irish paediatricians about Williams Syndrome patients and the WSAI. Ann and Kathleen were talking to parent support groups for other conditions (e.g. Cystic Fibrosis) for advice and guidance as to how to set up a support association. On November 9, 1986 Ann Breen wrote me concerning the definite progress she and Kathleen were making, but stated their anxiety about getting the WSAI established if not enough families responded.

No further correspondence was exchanged until 17½ months later when I got a letter (with letterhead of Williams Syndrome Association of Ireland) written March 16, 1988 by Ann Breen stating "we are still making slow but sure progress." Evidently the response had been less than Ann and Kathleen had hoped. The WSAI at that time was mostly trying to publicise itself and had been sending information about Williams Syndrome to families with newly diagnosed children, particularly newborns. It was not a terribly positive letter, but Ann's daughter, Karen, had shown much improvement and Ann seemed very positive about that.

Even by December 11 1989, the WSAI had not been approved as a charitable organisation (letter of April 5th, 1990 reiterated same) by the Irish Revenue Commissioners. Ann's frustration came out when she wrote; "it was nine (nine underlined twice) months before the application was processed. I will have to keep after them!" Unfortunately, most newly formed parent support groups go through these bureaucratic barriers which further complicates a long tedious process. I am also involved closely with three other parent support groups (Noonan Syndrome, Prader-Willi Syndrome, Charge Association) and they have experienced similar problems.

I was planning to attend a genetic conference in Manchester, England in September 1990 so Ann invited me to stop in Ballinasloe and talk to the WSAI. Was I surprised and pleased with the turnout for my talk on Williams Syndrome on September 27th, 1990. The WSAI group numbered at least 50 and they made me feel very good about my meagre efforts to assist the WSAI. I stayed at Ann's house and was able to play golf with her husband, Paschal and enjoy Karen and Mark.

Ann has never let me forget that I got her into starting the WSAI and that I am responsible for all the work it takes to keep the WSAI running. I do feel guilty, but every rare/uncommon "orphan" syndrome needs a support group and I don't know any other way to deal with the needs of the affected children and their families. Ann keeps me informed about all the WSAI activities and she has visited me and my family at our home in Lexington, Kentucky since the company she works for, Square D, has offices in Lexington. We trade Christmas cards each year with newsworthy comments and photographs.

Williams Syndrome got a big boost in 1993 when researchers localised the genes (at least 17, including the elastin gene) that cause the physical features and medical problems to chromosome number 7 on the long arm (7q11.23). It represents what we call a contiguous gene deletion syndrome. Some adult Williams individuals have had affected Williams Syndrome offspring suggesting that they are at a 50% risk of having similarly affected offspring because these 17 or so deleted genes are either not passed on (offspring unaffected) or the chromosome with the deleted genes is passed on (affected offspring). The elastin gene among these 17 or so genes is responsible for the heart defects, particularly the supravalvular aortic stenosis. All the remaining deleted genes have an adverse effect on facial development, mental potential, personality, growth, calcium metabolis and more.

My interest in Williams Syndrome is not limited to its unique patterning or physical development. The children have jerked my heartstrings in every possible way. I saw my first Williams case in June 1968. She was beautiful with lattice blue eyes, satellite hair, ruby red full lips, a coarse sexy voice, a wonderful smile and a warmness that immediately put me at ease. Their characteristic facial gestalt not only allows for instant diagnosis but also imparts to me the magic of nature's creativity. They are the special of the special and I enjoy being around them. I've diagnosed and followed approximately 60 cases in my career and I've learned from and greatly appreciated every single one of them. They are my favourites!

I'm sure this book of family stories will be a delightful roller coaster of emotions for everyone who reads it. There may be some sadness to it but, knowing these remarkable children and their families, it will set the stage for understanding and hope. I feel humbled and honoured to have been asked to pen its introduction.

Bryan D Hall, MD
Emeritus Professor of Paediatrics
University of Kentucky
Lexington
USA

My Story I

As I WALKED ALONG the long colourless hospital corridor once again I wondered for the umpteenth time—why me! Why me? Why did this have to happen to my child? After two and a half years to be told that my beautiful little daughter was "handicapped"? How could I accept this? To be told she has a condition that I had never heard of? What is Williams Syndrome anyway? That is what I want to know. I looked at her walking beside me. She does not look any different to the way she looked yesterday, yet everything is different now. "She will have an IQ of 56" the doctor told me. "Here is some information on her condition." I look at what she is handing me. It is a photocopied page from a medical textbook. It has some horrible black and white pictures on it. This is not my child! Someone has made a mistake! But even as I think that, I know in my heart it is not true. Karen is handicapped. Karen has Williams Syndrome! How will I tell her father? I cannot tell him on the phone. Today is only Monday and he will not be in Dublin with us until the weekend. Long days stretch in front of me. How can I ignore this news until Friday? Karen and I continue our journey along the white corridor. Just then I see Lillian and her mother come towards us. I remember! Lillian has just had her surgery to remove a cancerous tumour from her chest cavity. She is not a casual hospital acquaintance. She is the same age as my Karen. She was born in the same hospital on the same night as Karen. She was such a big healthy baby. I cannot believe she has this dreadful disease and that she is so sick. Her mother and I have not met since that time two and a half years ago in the maternity unit of our local hospital. Now here we both are in the hospital with our sick babies. The prognosis for Lillian is good. The chest tumour is usually the secondary stage of this particular cancer. However, for Lillian, it is the only stage. She has no other tumours and the doctors are very confident that the operation has been a success. Her mother is very hopeful for her future. Am I hopeful for Karen's future?

I settled Karen in her room and much later I left the hospital. I drove to my uncle's house. My uncle and his wife have been so supportive to us since Karen was born. This is not her first visit to the hospital in Dublin. How many times have I stayed here in this house over the last two and a half years? How many times have I headed to hospitals with Karen since she was born? The local paediatrician was very good to us when Karen was ill (as she was frequently). He always took care of her. He would take her to the hospital at a moments notice, sometimes just to give me a night's sleep! Karen did not sleep much at night as an infant. She cried at night, every night for about nine months. In the beginning I used to hold her, rock her, talk to her as she cried. Nothing I did made any difference. I even tried to get her to use a soother or dummy, something I always hated to see babies use. It made no difference. She just cried and cried, throwing up intermittently during the crying. I changed her sheet and her clothes many times each night. Eventually, I just sat with her, changing her sheet and clothes when necessary, and read books. I got through many "Mills and Boon" books during that long nine months of nights. I could read one a night! I have never been able to read a "Mills and Boon" book since!

Karen was very familiar with hospitals both at home and in Dublin. This latest visit to Dublin was "our last hope" to try to find out what was wrong with her. We had spent two and a half years hearing the doctors tell us "she is not normal but let us fix this problem first, then we will see." She had a lot of "problems" to be fixed and as soon as one was fixed we had to deal with the next one. Eventually I told the doctor that I needed to know what was wrong with her and we were referred to Dublin again as a "last hope." I really had not expected to get any answers this time either. After all we had been down this road many times already. Why should this time be any different? I sat in my room and thought—why had I demanded to know? Maybe I was better off yesterday when I only had a sick child. Yesterday I still had hope that she would get better, that she would be ok. Now I had a handicapped child who would never be "better." She would never be…I realised that I did not know what she would "never be." I did not know what she would be. I could not think of this any more. I had to get back to the hospital. I needed to see Karen, to be sure that she had not changed since yesterday. I somehow expected that she would look different or behave differently now that she was a different child. She was now a handicapped child. I got to her cot as quickly as I could. Her sweet smile met me as usual. I had always marvelled at that smile that could melt my heart. I took her in my arms and hugged her. She was not different! She would never be different to me. She would always be my baby!

Then the questions began to flow into my head. Karen has Williams Syndrome! Why us? Why did this have to happen to us? What do we do about it? What caused it? Was it something I did or didn't do? Is there any cure? Questions and more questions. No answers.

The days and nights that followed were very hard. Karen was as she had always been. However, things would never be the same for me again. Tuesday came. The doctors came to me and asked me if they could use Karen as a test case for the consultant's examinations that week. I agreed. I would sit by her cot and answer all the questions put to me without mentioning Williams Syndrome. I think I was on autopilot. On Wednesday I spoke to my aunt and uncle and told them about Karen's diagnosis. They had difficulties of their own at that time but all that was put to one side as they took in my news about Karen. We talked, cried and then talked and cried some more. It was such a relief to tell someone but it also made the whole situation harder to bear. Now that I had spoken about it to someone else it was somehow more real. There could be no more hope of Karen being a "normal" daughter. That was the hardest to bear. How I hated that word "handicapped." What did it mean anyway? I did not know anything about Williams Syndrome. Did the doctors know? I would ask them tomorrow. I did not! The next day I just sat with Karen and tried to believe that she was still the same child I had taken to the hospital! Well, she was, wasn't she? She looked the same, she behaved the same, she had the same difficulties she always had. But, no, she had one more thing now! She now had a label that said Williams Syndrome. Why, oh why had I insisted on finding out what was wrong with her? Why had I not left well enough alone? We could have managed. I would have looked after her and made her well. No, I would not have been able to do that! I was driving myself crazy. It is Thursday night. I have to pull myself together and get ready to break the terrible news to Karen's father tomorrow.

I did not sleep much that night either. I got up on Friday morning, had breakfast and went to the hospital. Karen was well and happy. I could almost forget the past week. I was somehow calm today. I think I felt that I had to be strong for Paschal today. This news was going to be a severe shock to him. After all, I had already had almost four days to get used to the idea of having a handicapped child. How would he take the news? He arrived in the afternoon. We spent some time with Karen and then left to go to my uncle's house. I told him in the car. I told him he had a daughter with Williams Syndrome and that I did not know what the future would hold for her or for us. He took the news very calmly. I think he had somehow known something already. Maybe I had not hidden my feelings as well as I thought during our phone calls this week. We sat in the car and held one another for quite a long time. We did not talk. There would be time enough for talking later. Right then we just needed to know that we would both be there for one another as well as for Karen. Maybe things would be all right after all! I closed my eyes and allowed my mind to drift back...

Karen's Story I

OUR DAUGHTER, KAREN, was born on 19th August 1983 after a normal pregnancy. My husband and I were thrilled that the baby was a girl as we already had a boy of 2 and a half years called Mark. Karen was small at birth weighing only 5 lbs. and 3 ozs. She also had an umbilical hernia and because of these two facts she was immediately taken to the hospital's special care baby unit. This meant that she was in an incubator for the first day and after that she continued to be looked after in the special care unit rather than the ordinary baby nursery.

We were reassured about this situation by the doctors and nurses. The doctor told us that the umbilical hernia was not unusual in newborn babies and that it would probably fix itself in time. They did not propose to do anything about it at that stage and they did not see her low birth-weight as a problem. I thought that it was due to the fact that I had a viral infection at approximately seven months in the pregnancy. During that time I had not put on any weight so I did not worry about the low birth-weight either. She did seem to have difficulty feeding and in keeping her bottle down. She was given very small amounts of formula at frequent intervals. After the usual number of days in the hospital I took Karen home.

I put her carrycot in our own bedroom as we had done with Mark. Her feeding difficulties continued and she began to suffer what was thought to be colic—she had a crying period in each 24 hours that usually started at 11 or 12 o'clock at night. She would then cry for between 3 and 5 hours at a time. After about three weeks I had to move Karen's cot out to the small bedroom as neither Paschal nor I was getting any sleep. I would sit on the spare bed by her cot watching to make sure that she did not suffocate on her own vomit as she tended to vomit during this time.

After the first few weeks I had discovered that holding her did not help her in any way and so, mostly, I just watched her and changed her sheets again and again. At her six-week check-up, the paediatrician felt that she might be suffering from a milk allergy and put her on Soya-bean based milk. He also prescribed medication for her in order to get her to sleep at night and "cry" during the day. This medication worked for about three nights and then she just reverted back to her old pattern. The Soya-bean based milk made no appreciable difference.

This situation persisted until Karen was about 9 months old. She refused any attempt to give her solid food and, despite many visits to the local hospital for observation and investigation, no one could pinpoint what Karen's problem was. I think some of her visits to the hospital were more for my benefit than for hers. At this stage, I was back at work and I was completely worn out due to lack of sleep and worry!! The doctor told me that she was not normal but could not tell me what was wrong with her. It was apparent at this stage that Karen's development was very slow. She was making no effort to walk and was not terribly interested in what was going on around her. I changed from full time to part time work because I felt that I could not cope any longer.

Then between 9 months and 12 months old things seemed to improve slightly. Karen's sleeping habits improved and I began to recover somewhat from the previous 9 months.

Paschal and I took a fortnight's holiday and my sister looked after Karen. This was a holiday that I was extremely glad to have had because otherwise I do not think I would have been able to cope with the ensuing months. We had barely returned from holiday (September 1984) when Karen developed a rectal prolapse. She had been prone to constipation and had shown a tendency towards prolapse since about six months of age. However, nothing could have prepared us for this situation. The rectum would prolapse about 3 inches, then become inflamed, swollen and bleeding. After the awful shock the first time it happened, I had to learn to cope with it. The doctors told me it was not causing Karen any pain and that it would correct itself when she got to 6 or 7 years of age. I was looking at Karen rolling around the floor in pain knowing there was nothing I could do for her.

At this time, she also became very listless and ill and vomited a lot of what I would describe as "brown vomit." It was blood stained mucous according to the doctors but they could not tell me what was causing it, even after extensive investigation in the local hospital. On release from hospital she contracted chicken pox and was extremely sick for a number of weeks. When she recovered from this she again suffered with the rectal prolapse and the vomiting.

She was referred to Our Lady's Hospital in Crumlin for investigation in November '84. The surgical team in Crumlin decided that she had, in fact, got two hernias rather than one umbilical hernia and that surgery was required straight away. This was done and Karen was released from the hospital in due course. However, no explanation for the vomiting had been found and nothing had been done to correct the rectal prolapse.

We had spent weeks in hospital again to no avail. I brought her back to Crumlin for her 6-week check-up after the surgery and, when her clothes were removed, she was covered in spots. I brought her home and called the doctor. Now she had measles—confluent measles as it turned out. She was so sick!

The doctor was afraid to send her to the local hospital in

case she might catch pneumonia because she would not have been strong enough to fight it. We cared for her at home and she made an extremely slow recovery over Christmas '84.

At this stage Karen was a year and a half old. She had had such a hard time since she was born that we felt that we hardly had time to get to know her as an individual. However, I did know one thing about her—she had a very loving smile and during the short periods of time when she was well, that loving personality had shone through. There were many nights when her little smile had saved her from my wrath—at 5 o'clock in the morning!

The feeding problems, the constipation, the rectal prolapse, the vomiting, all continued over the following months. The rectal prolapse was now so bad that something had to be done about it. Numerous trips to hospital, both Ballinasloe and Dublin, followed. Various different methods were tried i.e. sutures, wires, a course of injections—one a month under general anaesthetic. Eventually a wire was inserted into Karen's anal opening in Ballinasloe hospital and, with the aid of copious doses of laxatives each day, this solved the problem of the rectal prolapse. This, at least, gave both Karen and us some respite. She still suffered with constipation and, at times, had to have rectal "wash-outs" in order to keep the wire in place.

In September 1985 Karen had been assessed by a psychologist with the Brothers of Charity and had been described as "significantly delayed." After that, a social worker began to call to the house once a week to work with Karen. I learned what work to do with her and spent time each afternoon at this. It was terribly frustrating at first because I was trying to do too much with her. I learned that Karen's concentration span was very limited and she could only work for 4–6 minutes at a time. She had so much to learn! She had been so ill all her life that she had not picked up the normal things that babies learn. She had to start practically from scratch. It was all very difficult. Also, she was still only eating baby food and she was almost 2 and a half at this stage. She had even been force-fed in Crumlin hospital at one stage but nothing worked. She would just vomit it all back up.

During the Christmas season in 1985, we took some time out to review Karen's situation and were very unhappy with what we saw. This was her third Christmas and she was still suffering. I brought her back to the local hospital on the 31st December 1985 and spoke to her paediatrician. I told him that we needed to know what was wrong with Karen. We did not care what we had to do or where we had to bring her. We would have taken her to Australia if necessary to get some answers.

We were suffering immeasurably looking at her every day not knowing what was wrong with her, if she was going to live or die, what was next round the corner for us? We had no answers and could not look forward to any kind of future with her. We were living from day to day and all of us were beginning to crack under the strain. Mark, our son, had received very little of his parent's attention since Karen was born so he too was suffering. The biggest problem at this stage was that we could not see what the future was to be. So yet again we were referred back to Our Lady's Hospital in Crumlin.

We checked in to the hospital in Crumlin on 19th January 1986. Karen was just 2 years and 5 months old. On Monday 27th January Karen was diagnosed as having Williams Syndrome. A lady doctor sat me down and gave me the diagnosis. I felt numb. Having waited so long to be told what was wrong with Karen, I could not take it in when it finally happened. I suppose I had always had a little hope that whatever was wrong could be fixed by medication and that I would have the perfect daughter I always wanted. I had not expected a "syndrome," especially one I had never heard of. The doctor explained some things about the condition to me. She told me Karen had a heart murmur, that she was mentally retarded; that her IQ would be about 56 and that the condition was very rare. She gave me a copy of a page from a textbook with pictures of Williams Syndrome children. It could only be described as horrible!

I was advised to contact my local mentally handicapped services for support when I returned home. I told nobody at home about the diagnosis until the following Friday when Paschal came to Dublin to see us. Karen had not yet been released from hospital, as there were further tests they wanted to do.

My Story II

...AND SO WE EVENTUALLY LEFT the hospital in Dublin and headed home to Ballinasloe once again. This homecoming was different to all the others. We now had our answers but what did they mean? We spent the next couple of months trying to come to terms with the situation. We tried to comfort each other and I cried a lot, particularly at night. I had returned to work after we came home from the hospital and during the day I coped reasonably well. However, the evening times and the nights were terrible. I suppose we became a little depressed by it all. We did not know where to turn for information on Williams Syndrome or how to handle the whole situation. We looked at our beautiful daughter and wondered what her future would be.

Then something happened that brought me out of my lethargy. My colleagues at work collected money and sent Karen and myself to Lourdes on a pilgrimage. It was not that I was particularly religious but the thought that all these people cared enough to do this for us made me realise that I had to pick myself up and get on with my life as it now was.

By the time we returned from Lourdes I had decided that I was going to do as much to help Karen as I possibly could!

In order to do this I had to find out as much information as I could about Williams Syndrome. But how could I do this? All I had was the photocopied page from the hospital. It did not tell us very much. I began to ask questions, to look for information from anyone I came across—doctors, nurses, anyone! But no one seemed to know anything much about Williams Syndrome or know of anyone else who had the condition.

Then, out of the blue, I got a phone call from a friend of mine—a former work colleague. She told me that she had been listening to the "Gay Byrne Hour" on radio that day and that a woman had rung the programme to say she had a son who had just been diagnosed with Williams Syndrome. She asked me "Isn't that what your Karen has?" She said this woman was trying to get in touch with any other families that had a Williams Syndrome child. I could not believe it! There was someone else who had a child with this condition! Surely this other family would have some helpful information to give us. I could barely wait for the following morning to contact the radio programme to get in touch with them. I was so elated that I hardly slept that night. Early next morning I called the radio programme. I explained what I wanted and left my name and telephone number. They said that they would pass it on to the other family in question.

And so I waited...But not for long...

That afternoon at 2.00pm I received a phone call from this other family. And then my hope faded again. This family were in the exact same position as ourselves. Their son had just been diagnosed as well and they did not know anything about the condition either. They had been hoping to get information on Williams Syndrome from us! What a disappointment! Now what could we do? Still there were now two families so, between us, surely we could find out something somewhere.

Then I had a thought. The company I worked for in Ballinasloe was a subsidiary of an American company. The Ballinasloe Company reported directly to Head Office in Lexington in Kentucky, USA. If I could not find out anything about Williams Syndrome in Ireland, maybe I could get some information from America. So I approached the Human Resources Manager in Ballinasloe and asked him to help me. He immediately contacted the Human Resources Manager in USA and within a very short time I had a response from the USA. I was given contact details for three different people that might be able to help me. Two of these contacts were people in Ireland that turned out to be false leads. However, the third contact was for Bryan Hall, a professor of genetics in the University of Kentucky in Lexington, USA. (Bryan was to become an invaluable source of information on WS and, I am proud to say, a life long friend). At that time, I wrote to him and sent him a detailed history of Karen.

Then I waited...not knowing if this was to be another false lead. Very quickly he wrote back saying that he was very familiar with Williams Syndrome, that it seemed fairly sure from the history that Karen did have the condition but that he would like to see photographs of her from birth to the present time in order to confirm the diagnosis. I could not believe it! I had finally managed to find someone who knew something about Williams Syndrome!

I rooted through the photograph albums and found a representative selection of pictures of Karen since she was born. I sent these to Bryan and waited again...I remember the morning I received the next letter from Bryan. I held it in my hand for a long long time before I opened it! It was like I was afraid to open it! I have never been quite sure why! After all, this was just confirmation, wasn't it? Somehow, it didn't seem like that. I think I was still hoping a little—that the doctors had got it wrong, that I might yet have my "normal" daughter. I opened the letter. The doctors had not gotten it wrong! There it was in black and white again. Karen had Williams Syndrome. Tears flowed and I could not read any further!

This is it then, isn't it? Karen has Williams Syndrome. So... the questions began to flow into my head again. Why us? Why did this have to happen to us? What do we do about it? What caused it? Was it something I did or didn't do? Is there any cure? Questions and more questions. This time, instead of accepting that I have no answers and feeling sorry for myself, I begin to wonder how or where I can find the answers. There have to be some answers somewhere. What about this professor in America? Surely he can help! I pick up his letter again and this time I force myself to read past the first sentence.

There it is—the first road I must travel to start finding the answers I so desperately need. This kind person, who does not know me, or anything about me, is offering to meet with my family in London in September of this year. He says he will be attending a conference in Manchester and plans to spend a few days in London as well. He will be very happy to meet with us and give us what information he can on Williams Syndrome. How wonderful! I could barely wait to show the letter to Paschal. There was no question in either of our minds about us making that trip in September. We were most certainly going!

I contacted Professor Hall and told him about the other Irish WS family and asked if they could accompany us to London for our meeting with him. This he readily agreed to. I contacted the other WS family and told them of the proposed trip. They were delighted and began to make plans to travel to London as well.

September 1986. Travel to London. What a time in our lives! We had spent the last couple of months building all our hopes on this trip that promised us so much. Surely this eminent professor from America would have all the answers! But he is an eminent professor! Why would he be interested in two Irish WS families? Is he really interested in helping us? Maybe he is just being polite and will not have much time to give us? Would we be disappointed?

We need not have worried. We were not disappointed. Bryan Hall could not have been more kind and gentle in his handling of two Irish families in the throes of anguish at the hand that life had suddenly dealt them. He patiently explained as much about Williams Syndrome as he felt we were able to cope with. He told us how beautiful our two WS children were. He pointed out the WS facial features, told us of the endearing personality WS people have, he said all the kind and positive things. He also, however, answered our straight questions with straight answers.

We ended up with an overall view of the WS condition tempered with the reminder that not all of the "parts" of WS would apply to our own children. He told us of the things to be aware of like the heart condition that can affect some people with Williams Syndrome, the kidney problems that can arise sometimes undetected, the difficulties experienced when teachers think our WS children understand more than they actually do and so on and so on. He told us so much!

And then he said something that planted a seed in my head that has germinated over the years. He said "Now there are your two families with a Williams Syndrome child in Ireland. There must be many more families out there going through the same anguish that you are experiencing. You need to start a WS parent support group in Ireland."

Such a simple sentence! I did not know it then but that sentence was to have a profound effect on my life and the lives of my family.

The WSAI Story I

"YOU SHOULD TRY TO SET UP a Williams Syndrome Parent Support Group in Ireland!" Professor Hall felt that there should be significant numbers of WS individuals in Ireland, probably a lot of whom were not diagnosed. He said we should try to get in contact with as many as possible. Yes, we decided, we would! At this point we were buoyed up with enthusiasm! This generous person from America had helped us so much already that we now wanted to pass on that help to all other Irish WS families!

But how does one go about such a venture?

After our meeting with Professor Hall finished, the two families spent some time together discussing all that we had learned. We were so happy to finally have found someone who knew about Williams Syndrome! We discussed the idea of forming a parent support group as had been suggested and we decided that together we would do it.

We travelled home to Ireland with renewed vigour for the challenges ahead. We did not expect life to be rosy! We still had our own learning disabled children to look after but we now felt that, with all the new information we had, we were ready to move forward.

And so began the process of forming a parent support group...

First: Professor Hall had told us that there was a Williams Syndrome Association in existence in the USA and that he would send me contact details for them. The contact details duly arrived and I wrote to them. I explained the situation regarding WS in Ireland and said that we were trying to start a parent support group. I asked for their help.

Second: We made contact with cardiologists, paediatricians and other medical people in Ireland to ask for their help and support.

Third: We tried to contact other WS families in Ireland. This was to be the difficult bit, of course! We decided to use the national radio station that had put our two families in contact originally. I wrote to The Gay Byrne Radio Programme and asked them to make an announcement for us. This they did and we got in touch with a few other WS families.

The WSA in America replied to my letter. They told me that they would give me whatever help they could. They also told me that there was an association in England that had helped them get their own association started. This association was called The Infantile Hypercalcaemia Foundation at that time (it is now known as the Williams Syndrome Foundation).

As a result of contact between USA and England I received a letter from Lady Cynthia Cooper of the UK WS Association in January '87. She gave me contact details for the Northern Ireland region of their association. I contacted them and received some very helpful literature on WS in February '87. More importantly, however, they sent me contact details for some other Irish WS families that had been in touch with them.

So...I now had a mailing list, be it ever so small!!!

I wrote to Bryan Hall in Kentucky to let him know of our progress.

Then I started to try to get the few WS families together, to meet, chat and exchange ideas. This proved to be very difficult. You must remember that the numbers were very small, the families were spread all around the country, most were leading very busy lives and also trying to rear a learning disabled child!

I tried to have the meetings on a Sunday to give people the best chance of being able to attend. Sometimes it worked, sometimes it didn't! Many, many times, arranged meetings had to be cancelled at the last minute. However, when the meetings did actually take place, the families seemed to get so much from them that we continued to persevere.

We were now heading into the summer of 1987 and I decided that I would put press releases in the national newspapers to announce the formation of the Williams Syndrome Association of Ireland (WSAI). I also hoped that we might find some more WS families. This, to me, was the official formation of the association!

Karen's Story II

AND SO WE BROUGHT KAREN HOME...

The doctor in Crumlin hospital had advised me to contact the local mentally handicapped services for support when I returned home. However, we had been in touch with them already because, even though we had not known what was wrong with Karen, we knew that something was! She had certainly not been developing as normal so we had already had her psychologically assessed. She had been referred to the Brothers of Charity and some early intervention had already begun for her.

On returning home, I contacted the local paediatrician who had been so helpful to me over the years since Karen was born. At that time he was not convinced of Karen's diagnosis of Williams Syndrome. I showed him the photocopied page from the medical textbook but he was not familiar with Williams Syndrome. He said he would try to get some information about it for me.

Karen at this stage was two and a half years old. She was reasonably ok medically. She had a heart murmur that needed monitoring and she was still suffering with constipation and rectal prolapse. Still, the immediate need was to find out what support services were available to us locally. The paediatrician referred Karen to the local Brothers of Charity consultant paediatrician and she was seen by her in February 1986. She checked her thoroughly but she could not tell us anything very much about Williams Syndrome.

From then on we began to get more visits from psychologists, nurses, social workers, etc. attached to the Brothers of Charity Services. A program of intervention was put together for Karen and we began the process of trying to help her learn. She was still in nappies, of course, and there was certainly no thought of trying to toilet train her then! She was still not eating any solid food—despite repeated efforts to get her to do so! They had even tried to force feed her in Crumlin hospital at one point with disastrous results. She just threw everything up so I refused to allow it to continue.

I began to feed her Complan at one point in order to supplement her bottle feeds and this worked very well. That is until there was some scare about Complan and it was removed from sale! I panicked! That food was what was keeping my daughter alive! I could not do without it! Thankfully, I had a very understanding pharmacist who gave me what stock was left in the shop. This kept us going for quite some time!

At this time, I was going to work from 9.30am to 1.30pm each day. My sister took care of Karen for me and I then spent time each afternoon working with Karen. The progress was very slow. Her level of concentration was very poor. I used flashcards with words on them to try to improve her vocabulary. I got some from the social worker and I also made my own from baby books. I had cards with all the letters of the alphabet as well as words. I had cards with the names of household items that I used to stick up around the house!

I found that we could work for a number of weeks and Karen did not seem to learn anything at all. She would know it while we were doing it but would have forgotten everything by the next day. It was very frustrating! Then I realised that one day she just knew it and remembered it! It was like it took time for the information to get into her "long term" memory. After that I did not get so frustrated with her. I just kept repeating things day after day and waited for the day when she would just know it and retain it. This did invariably happen. It seemed to take about three months work. I have continued to notice this pattern in her learning over the years.

The Brothers of Charity offered a preschool placement for Karen when she was about three and a half years old. This placement was from 10.00am to 1.30pm for 5 days a week. She settled in there very well. However there was one big problem—Karen's feeding. She was still not taking any solid food. She was existing on Baby Milupa along with her bottle. I had managed to get her from the Complan drink to the Milupa foods.

The manager of the preschool decided that she had to eat regular food and tried to insist that she eat her dinner. I did not realise this at first until I arrived to collect Karen one day and found her still sitting at the table with a plate of cold dinner in front of her! I asked what was going on and was told. Needless to say, that regime did not continue! I complained vociferously and that situation never occurred again.

Still Karen had a feeding difficulty that had to be addressed. It did take a long time and a lot of hard work but eventually we got her to eat solid food. It was a joint effort between us at home and the staff at the preschool. We just very gradually introduced new foods into Karen's diet. Actually, calling it a diet is misleading! For example she had Milupa every morning—never anything else! We gradually introduced a tiny piece of weetabix into the Milupa. I do mean a tiny piece—a pinch!

Over a very long period of time the Milupa became totally weetabix and she then ate weetabix for breakfast for months and years afterwards. She was never one for a varied diet! She would never eat sweets, ice-cream, desserts, etc. I have often wondered what the casual onlooker thought when they saw me go into a shop and buy ice-creams for myself, Paschal and Karen's brother, Mark while Karen sat there without anything! It must have looked extremely odd!

Karen remained in the preschool until she was six years of age. She was monitored all during her time there by the psychologist. Then a decision had to be made about where she would go next. The options were a centre for the severely disabled in Ballinasloe, a special school for the moderately disabled in Athlone or the local primary school.

Well, there was no real decision! The only question was— which placement suited Karen's abilities best. Thankfully, at that time, there was no disagreement on the issue. Everyone working with Karen agreed that the special school in Athlone was where she should go.

So, that was where she went. She was collected by bus each morning at about 8.00am and delivered home again at about 3.00pm. She progressed very well in the school within her ability level and she liked being there, which was the most important thing.

It was during her time there that I saw one of the traits of Williams Syndrome stand out. I had liaised very closely with Karen's first teacher when she started in the school. I explained Williams Syndrome to her and gave her as much information as I could. That was fine and everything worked well. Then, after a year or two, Karen was moved to the next class and a new teacher. I knew this was happening but thought it should be fine. And it was! Far too fine! I began to get glowing reports on Karen's progress from her new teacher. I could not believe that she was talking about my Karen! I investigated! The new teacher was accepting every "Yes" answer that Karen gave her! She did not realise that Karen would answer "Yes" to any question she did not understand or, sometimes, just did not want to bother answering! So, every time the teacher asked her did she understand something she said "Yes" and the teacher believed her!

Hence my spectacular daughter! I realised later on that this is a difficulty with Williams Syndrome. The language skills and verbal abilities of children with Williams Syndrome can lead those working with them to assume that they are better and more able than they actually are!

As I said already, Karen enjoyed the special school. Her friendly and outgoing personality endeared her to the staff. However, as with most WS children, she did not relate very well to the other students. She preferred to deal with the adults i.e. the staff!

It was during her time in the special school that she first got involved with Special Olympics. The school always took part in the Special Olympics competitions and Karen first participated in gymnastics. To my surprise, she was quite good at gymnastics! Because of the poor hand eye coordination associated with WS, I had expected that she would find gymnastic routines very challenging. She did not and went on to win a number of medals.

It was not long, however, before swimming became her Special Olympic sport. Since she was very young, her father and I had taken her and Mark to the local swimming pool in Ballinasloe. She loved the water and moved readily from shallow end to deep end with her armbands on. When we eventually took the armbands off she still wanted to move freely from shallow end to deep end! And after a few scary moments (for us, not her!) she did just that. I quickly understood that there was no distinction for her—it was all deep as far as she was concerned! And swimming seemed to come naturally to her.

She began to take part in Special Olympics swimming galas and began to win medals there too! Eventually she would go on to represent Ireland at the Special Olympics European Games in Holland in 2000. There she won gold, silver and a fourth place ribbon.

And so we gradually moved from having a sick handicapped child to having a European Gold Medal Winner in our home! How strangely the wheels of life turn!

Sorry, I am getting ahead of myself!

Karen continued in her special school until she was eighteen years old. Those were not easy years by any means. We had ongoing checkups, visits to psychologists, visits from social workers, visits from nurses, etc.,etc.,etc. Her general health was reasonable good during these years but her heart murmur had to be monitored and she had to have annual kidney tests done.

As a young girl with an outgoing and friendly personality we had the worries of how to keep her safe from harm. I remember attending a meeting locally when Karen was about seven or eight. There was a visiting psychologist there to give advice to the families on various different issues. I asked his advice on how to protect my daughter from strangers in the years ahead.

At that stage I was trying to allow Karen a certain amount of freedom to explore the neighbourhood and still keep her safe. The advice I was given, after a lengthy discussion, was that I should give her a list of the names of the people that she was allowed to speak to! This was so ludicrous that it dented my faith in psychologists for a long time afterwards! Imagine! Give a list of names to a child who could not even read, who was known by more people locally than I was myself, who knew people that I did not know! What nonsense! Obviously, that psychologist had never reared a child!

One of the things that we noticed in Karen from a very early age was a fear of certain noises. This fear of noises, we eventually discovered, was due to the hyperacusis that is part of the Williams Syndrome condition. She couldn't tolerate the hoover being used in the house for a long number of years. She did eventually get used to that noise and now it does not bother her at all. However, there are still some noises that she cannot tolerate e.g. food processor, food mixer on high speed, etc.

She also loved to watch the washing machine at work. She would (and still does!) sit for a long time watching it. I eventually realised that it was not the "watching" that was the attraction for her! It was the "listening"! I realised it was the sound the machine was making, particularly during the spin cycle, that attracted her.

This "sound" attraction also manifests itself in her love of visiting airports. One of the things she likes to do is to go to the airport in Dublin. Her father brings her and they park the car on a roadside near the airport. There she loves to watch/ listen to the planes taking off. The planes landing do not have the same interest at all! Again, I believe, it is the engine sound that is piquing her interest!

She also loves to listen to foreign language programmes on TV and particular parts of films that have interesting or different sounds.

The most obvious evidence of this interest in "sounds" is, of course, Karen's love of music. This was evident from a very early age although we did not realise how keen that interest was for quite some time. Looking back, it is obvious now that almost from the day she was born, Karen loved music. Even as an infant, music would soothe her when she was sick or upset. I remember playing tapes for her in the kitchen when she was small and she would just gravitate towards the music.

Very soon birthday presents and Christmas presents became "something musical." If anyone asked what to get her as a present they were told "something musical." The house filled up with musical things—toy keyboards, tape players, little musical toys, etc.

Eventually, when she was about seven years old, we bought a full size Casio keyboard for her. The thing was far too big for her at the time—she could hardly reach the keys—but I wanted something that was safe and sturdy for her to use. It had a very secure stand and there was no danger of it falling over on her.

So she began to play this keyboard! At first I thought she was just making "noise" with it but very quickly the "noise" changed to music. I began to pay more attention and I realised that she was actually playing music. I watched her while she listened to some tune on Top of the Pops on BBC and then went to the front room and played the same tune on her keyboard! I was fascinated!

About 1994/1995, I began to read some interesting things in the magazine from the Williams Syndrome Association in the USA. They were just discovering that some Williams Syndrome people had a special musical ability. They had started a music camp for a week in the summer to foster this musical ability. I began to wonder more about Karen's musical ability then. However, we were at a disadvantage in our home because the rest of us there were not particularly musical. Karen was the only one who was! We decided that we needed to find out if she really had musical ability and if she had, we had to help her develop it!

The WSAI Story II

SUMMER 1987. The press releases have appeared in the national newspapers. Now there is an official Williams Syndrome Association of Ireland! However, there are only 6 or 7 families involved. Our main task is still to try to contact more WS families. We believe that there should be at least 150 families in the south of Ireland.

I now have letter headed paper for the association and we are very delighted to be able to name The Right Honourable Desmond Guinness as the Patron of the association. A meeting of doctors, social workers and a couple of parents was held at his home to discuss what we were trying to do and to see if it was worthwhile. We all thought it was and this kind gentleman then agreed to be our patron to help us in our work.

I am now in regular contact with the Infantile Hypercalcaemia Foundation (IHC) in the UK and also their regional co-ordinator in the North of Ireland, both of whom have been of immense help to me in getting our own association up and running. We have been trying to get publicity for the association but we appear to be in a "catch 22" situation—

nobody wants to know because they have never heard of us!!

Still we persevere and 1987 rolls on into 1988. I write to Professor Bryan Hall to give him an update on our progress. Even reading that letter again today I can see the underlying air of pessimism in it! I really did not see that this association was ever going to get anywhere worthwhile. Many times during these early years I made a conscious decision to forget about it and concentrate on doing the best I could for Karen and the rest of my own family! After all, who was I to think I could start an association of any sort!

But then I would get one more phone call or letter from another WS family and my energy was renewed. I used to think "if I can help even one family not to have to endure the heartache I had endured in the first few years of Karen's life then it will have been worthwhile."

It was at the start of September 1988 that I received a letter from a family in Galway. It was a long letter detailing the first two years of life of a boy with Williams Syndrome. I read the letter over and over. I felt I could have just changed the boy to a girl called "Karen" and practically all of the information in that letter would have remained true.

The boy's name was Alan.

Alan's Story

I BECAME PREGNANT WITH OUR FIRST CHILD in October 1985 and my husband and I were both delighted. I gave up work and stayed at home. Alan was born in August 1986. He was ten days overdue, he weighed 3.360 kg and he was a normal delivery. I thought he was very greasy and had a lot of hair on his head and on his body. The nurses assured me that once he was washed and dressed he would look ok, which he did.

I breast fed him for the first two days but he did not want to breast feed. The day after he was born he was examined by a paediatrician. He told me that Alan had a heart murmur, that one of his testes was un-descended and that he had infection in both his eyes. When he cried he had a very hoarse cry and any sudden noise in the ward seemed to startle him.

We took him home and I continued to breast feed him. He was not a very settled baby. He was anxious and did not sleep very well. At five weeks he started to cry a lot and he was very unsettled. I took him to the doctor who said that he had colic. He gave me medication to put in his feeds, this did not help. This continued and Alan seemed to be getting worse. He was always pulling his legs up to his body when he cried and seemed to be in pain. I brought him to casualty and they said he had an inguinal hernia. They kept him in overnight and operated on him the next morning. He was released the next day.

I continued to breast feed him after he came home. The following week the same problems occurred again—the crying and pulling his legs up towards his body. He seemed very uncomfortable. I took him back to my GP who said he had another hernia on his other side. He was sent back into hospital and had his second hernia repaired. He came home from hospital and was ok for a few days.

I then began bottle feeding Alan. He took his bottle at night time and was a much happier baby. After a few months he was checked by the public health nurse. She did not think he was progressing as normal and he had an ear infection the day she visited. He had begun teething. He was now four or five months old. He continued to bottle feed. He did not seem to be making any progress at this stage and this caused me concern. I consulted my paediatrician who assured me he was doing fine and that his weight was ok. I went home very frustrated. I started to feed Alan a little baby rice. He was happy taking that for a few weeks then he would just vomit all over the place.

Both my husband and I felt that Alan should be doing more at six months of age. We continued to talk to the doctors who said he was doing fine. As the months progressed Alan continued to get anxious, he was continuously crying, not sleeping at night, vomiting and constipated. We went back to the doctors who treated him for constipation. At nine months, he was not drinking much and eating less! He was just lying in his cot listless and, when he was put sitting up, he had to be supported by cushions. I noticed that his urine was strong smelling and took him to the doctor. The doctor checked his urine and Alan was treated for a kidney infection but showed no signs of improvement.

The paediatrician told me that I was a fussy mother and I had a fussy child and just to continue doing what I was doing with him. I tried to stimulate him by helping him to look at picture books, read nursery rhymes and play with soft toys but this did not work. At ten months I noticed that Alan was not taking much fluids and, aware that he could get dehydrated, I brought him to my GP. Alan was admitted into hospital again where he remained for three weeks. During this time urine, blood, kidney tests and bone scans were carried out. Alan was sent home as they could not find anything wrong with him. At eleven months I was contacted by the hospital as they had noticed something on the recent x-rays that was different to his previous x-rays. Alan was again admitted to hospital and remained there for three weeks. He weighed 16lbs and was eleven months old. He did not respond to anything except noise. He started crying when any noise was made around him. The tests concluded that Alan had infantile hypercalcaemia. The nurses tried to feed Alan with liquidised potato and carrot but he vomited soon after. They also tried pureed apple.

He was referred to a dietician, who said Alan would have to maintain a low calcium diet and would have to avoid vitamin D and sunlight. Alan did not respond well to the low calcium diet. He was still constipated, irritable and did not gain weight. The dietician assured me it would take some time for his calcium levels to return back to normal but that when they did he would make good progress. He was put on a formula called Locasol which he seemed to tolerate well—no vomiting.

I contacted the company who produced Locasol. They sent me information consisting of two sheets outlining why the product was prescribed to children. It was prescribed for children with hypercalcaemia and also for another more severe form where the child had very small facial features, heart and kidney problems and a mental handicap. I asked the paediatrician about this information and he said he believed that Alan did not suffer from this. He felt that once his calcium levels returned to normal he would be ok. I believed him and hoped this would happen.

Alan returned from hospital. He had made some progress as he was drinking his bottles again but was still crying. His kidney infections had abated but he was still unable to do any of the things a normal one year old child could do e.g. he was unable to walk or talk. Slowly but surely I saw some progress in Alan. He began to notice things in the house and pay more attention. However, he still had only managed to eat small amounts of liquidised potato and carrot and pureed apple and he never seemed hungry.

At this stage I asked the paediatrician if he could check out Alan's heart condition. He had an echocardiogram done and they said his heart murmur was very slight. Alan continued to make some progress and began to eat larger portions of varied liquidised foods. His calcium levels decreased and he seemed more content.

He began to walk at twenty one months. His movements were quite awkward and his legs crossed over one another. He had a problem sleeping at night but he never seemed tired. Alan was put in his own bed but he left this and wandered around the house regularly. He was afraid of rain on the window and thunder. Alan was unable to speak but he listened to the television and enjoyed music. He was now walking and sleeping better.

From three months to two years Alan was constantly vomiting after each feed and crying for hours on end. When he cried his two big blue eyes looked at you pleadingly, asking you to do something for the discomfort he was in.

I still wanted to obtain further information regarding infantile hypercalcaemia. I asked the paediatrician were there any other children in Galway or Ireland with this condition The paediatrician gave me contact details for two other people with a similar child. That was in August 1988. I contacted Ann Breen and told her my story.

Dear Mrs Breen,

I have a boy of two who has been diagnosed as having Ideopathic Hypercalcaemia since last July '87. My paediatrician at the Regional Hospital gave me some addresses, yours included, to get in touch with you.

My name is Nuala and my husband's name is Michael and Alan is our first child, born August 4th, 1986.

At birth he had a slight heart murmur. This is still present slightly and he has a check-up with a cardiologist every 6–9 months. It was a normal delivery, 10 days overdue. I was very well all through the pregnancy.

I breast fed him for the first few weeks. At 5 weeks old he had terrible pain. I took him to my G.P. who said it was colic. The crying lasted for 2 hours at times throughout the day. The doctor gave me Gaviscon sachets to put through his feed so I had to introduce bottle and teat then. The crying and pain remained. One night it was so bad I took him to the hospital where they said he had a left inguinal hernia. They kept him in and operated. He was fine after that until a week later he had the right side operated on for a hernia also.

After that he was full bottle fed on SMA Gold Cap formula. He got bad colic. The paediatrician changed the food to Wysoy (Soya bean based milk) which made him very constipated at three months. That was changed to Cow & Gate. He would be ok for 2 weeks and then get colic again. No medication was of any use. At 4 months he was put on Pregestarril. He was again ok for 2 weeks and then back to the colic! I, myself, put him on cow's milk and he seemed ok on that. I thought my problems were over!

At 6 months he got an ear infection due to teething.

At 8 months he was 23 lbs weight, still on the milk but not progressing or sitting up or doing any of the normal things. The paediatrician said he was ok.

At 9 months he got a kidney infection and constipation lasting 2—3 days. My G.P. gave me baby enema which was of no use either. I used to give him bottles of sugar and water and I used to try to evacuate his bowel manually which was terrible!

He wasn't great at eating at any stage but then he started to refuse spoon feeds and he'd vomit up everything, even the bottles. He seemed to get relief then. He started losing weight and at 10 months he only weighed 19 lbs. My G.P. couldn't know what was wrong! Alan was almost all the time constipated and the doctor gave me Colace to soften the stools. That was of no use either. He kept getting kidney infections and also vomiting most of the bottles.

Then the G.P. referred me back to the paediatrician. Alan was admitted to hospital. They did every test on him for bloods, urine, faeces, 24 hour urine collection, x-rays, I.V.P. The only thing that showed was a raised blood urea and the I.V.P. didn't show anything.

He was sent home not having any idea what was wrong saying that he was a fussy child, was making himself sick and that I was too anxious and that I'd have to force him to eat! His diet was changed to Nutramagen instead of milk. He still lost weight down to 16 lbs and was also constipated. He was constipated for 10 days.

A few days later they contacted me from the hospital saying that the radiologist had noted a change in his bone structure from previous x-rays.

He was admitted again. This time they did a calcium blood test and discovered that it was over the normal -3.90 it was, they said. That was at 11 months.

The paediatrician then said that all the previous problems were all to do with this Hypercalcaemia. The dietician then visited me and gave me a diet sheet of calcium and vitamin D free food. She also said to give him Locasol to drink.

He remained in hospital for 3 weeks on that diet. He was so sick that he just lay there listless. He was very reluctant to eat again and it was a hard 3 weeks feeding him. He began to drink better. Eventually the blood calcium lowered slightly and he was allowed home.

He has been having 2 monthly check-ups since.

It was very frustrating coping with him from then until now! He still refused to eat and made himself sick. Everything had to be liquidised and still has. He'd drink his bottle very well.

He slowly improved. The constipation was over (and the kidney infections) at last. By 16 months he could move about in the walker. He took an interest in things. He started walking at 21 months.

He has no speech yet except his own mumble of words. He doesn't feed himself. I'm starting potty training. He sleeps better and has few pains

I've probably forgotten lots of things to tell you. Hope this letter doesn't bore you too much.

Is there anyone who can give me more information about the problem as I have been given very little about it?

Thank you for reading this.
Looking forward to a reply from you soon.
Yours sincerely

Nuala

I quickly received a letter from Ann containing information about Williams Syndrome. I returned to my paediatrician and asked him if my son had Williams Syndrome. At this stage he confirmed that he had. I then asked what help was out there for Alan. He said he would put me in contact with the Brothers of Charity who dealt with learning disabilities.

A social worker came to the house and met both Michael and I and outlined the procedures followed for children with learning disabilities. A psychologist came to the house and talked us through the program they would work on with Alan. A nurse and a paediatrician from the Brothers of Charity worked with us over the following years.

Alan's calcium levels were continuously monitored and he had begun to eat some solid food. The Brothers of Charity provided excellent support and taught Alan basic things like learning to sit at a table for a short while although his concentration was very poor. They also worked on his hand and eye coordination. Over a period of six months we eventually got Alan into a pattern of sleeping in his bed on his own. This was a huge achievement. He was two and a half at this stage. He was still very sensitive to sudden sounds.

I met Ann Breen in late 1988 and I met her daughter, Karen. I continued to meet Ann over the years. It was great to talk to someone who understood what we were going through. I became involved with the Williams Syndrome Association of Ireland.

When Alan was three he became very irritable again and cried a lot. Tests proved inconclusive. I found a lump in Alan's stomach and believed it was a hernia. Alan was operated on, the surgeon noticed the muscles over his stomach area were very lax and sutured them together. Since then Alan has not had any problems with hernias and his eating has greatly improved.

The Brothers of Charity suggested enrolling him in a preschool two days a week to start with, although he was unable to speak. He went two days a week and seemed to enjoy this. Alan was not toilet trained at this stage. When he was three and a half he went to a preschool with the Brothers of Charity where he had the benefit of both Occupational and Speech Therapy and a Psychologist.

When I received all the information from Ann regarding Williams Syndrome, I did not know what to think. I was on my own when I received the letter. I felt relieved in a way but also angry and upset as to why this had happened to us and the lack of information from the professionals. I read the literature again and cried as I did so. I was not prepared to read that mental handicap was a feature of this condition. I could not accept that and wondered why. Michael came home from work and we read the letter again. He was speechless for a while and very emotional but said we will deal with this problem together and contact Ann again to find out all we can to help this baby of ours. We talked to our families about it and they also found it hard to understand. I had never worked with a child with disabilities before even though I was a nurse. I wondered how people would deal with Alan; would they stop and stare.

Both Michael and I knew how difficult it was to live with Alan. However, some family members who had not spent much time with Alan felt we were overreacting. My family wondered where it came from. Michael and I did not always discuss the issue. Sometimes there was just silence; this was putting a strain on our marriage. I was at home all day with Alan and did not seem to get any break. We went out occasionally at night time but Alan always seemed to be unwell when we were gone. My husband's family lived locally and they would help out whenever they could.

I decided that I would go back to work as I could not stay at home all the time. I got an evening job. This was a new lease of life for me and it enabled me to cope better with Alan. Anyone I talked to about Williams Syndrome had never heard of it.

Alan continued to attend pre-school two days a week and special pre-school two days a week. Transport was provided for him. He had a habit of sticking tissues up his nose; he had to be taken to hospital three times due to this to have them removed under anaesthetic. Around this time I noticed a problem with his eyes as he would not look straight at objects. He was referred to an eye specialist who noted that he had a squint and said that he would have to have his eyes patched each day for a few hours. He said he did not require glasses. His eyes were patched for two hours a day for the next three years. This was very difficult as I had to sit with him and restrain him as otherwise Alan would pull the patch off. However, the patches did rectify the problem.

His appetite improved a lot but when eating solid foods he did not seem to chew. He swallowed everything whole! He was still given the Locasol each day and his calcium levels were monitored once a year. He was not toilet trained but was aware of having to wear a nappy. We began potty training. This was a slow process but we succeeded. By the time he was six years of age Alan was fully toilet trained.

Our second son, Jason, was born in 1991.

The speech therapist worked out a program for Alan so we could work with him at home; he had to match up pictures, blow bubbles, make all types of sounds and pretend play to encourage words and sentences. He loved to be outside running around. He was unable to kick a football but enjoyed running in the wind. He did not like walking on anything higher than the ground e.g. stairs, etc.

He did not have any fear of strangers and was very friendly with anyone he met. Alan had a fascination with anything that spun—he would watch the washing machine going through a full cycle. Any toys he had with wheels he spun them around.

With regard to Alan's medical problems, the cardiologist told us that the type of heart murmur Alan had was atrial septal defect and he also had pulmonary stenosis which would be monitored regularly. His kidney infections had stopped, but his kidneys were still monitored every two years in case he had calcium deposits in his kidneys due to his high calcium levels earlier on. He got a chest infection when he was four and a half. He was hospitalised with bronchitis and was given medication that resulted in him becoming very hyperactive. This was very difficult to deal with. The doctors assured me that this was unrelated to Williams Syndrome.

Alan was hospitalised twice more with suspected bronchitis. On his third visit to hospital he was diagnosed with asthma and associated allergies.

Alan did not have any problems when his baby teeth were falling out. The new tooth pushed the baby tooth out of the way as normal. His hair stood up on the top of his head and could not be styled any particular way. His lower lip hung out and he dribbled a lot. We had to remind him to suck his lip in. At play school he loved to play tin whistle and the mouth organ.

By the age of four he began to speak and he did not stop! He was able to tell us everything. I noticed that Alan made sure he knew his words 100% before he learned new words. He also imitated people and used phrases that he did not understand. He was very tuned in to people's feelings. We were beginning to see Alan the child rather than Alan with Williams Syndrome. He was beginning to develop his own personality. We now looked forward to his childhood as we felt we were able to deal with Alan and he was progressing well. As his brother grew up he was able to do lots of things Alan had just started to do. They were good company for each other and Alan learned a lot from his younger brother.

By the time Alan was six years old we had to review his education. We met with the psychologist, the social worker, the nurse and the speech therapist. We were told they thought it best that Alan was enrolled into a special school. We had mixed feelings about this as we thought he could continue to go to the special school and also attend the local national school. We were told this was not an option as the Department of Education did not accommodate children with special needs in this way.

He commenced schooling in the special school. Some pupils in his class were unable to speak. Alan found this very frustrating and he came home from school in a temper and was not progressing. After two weeks I was not happy with the situation and consulted the social worker suggesting that Alan be enrolled in the local primary school to see how he would get on.

The principal of the local primary school was prepared to take Alan for one year to see how he would fit in. Alan attended the primary school for one year. He may not have learnt a lot at the school, but he gained valuable social skills and was able to mix with the other children. We reviewed this with the psychologist who believed that Alan should be enrolled in another special school, one that might be more suited to his needs. In 1993, Alan began attending the school where he remained until he was eighteen years old.

Alan was fully toilet trained, his eating and sleeping patterns were very good and he got on well with his brother. He enjoyed playing outside and he had begun to learn how to swim. On one occasion my sister brought him to the circus but he ran away as he was terrified by the noise.

At school he took part in everything—reading, writing, swimming, nature walks, cookery and PE. Alan's concentration was still very poor but he learnt to read and write at a very basic level. He got very involved with swimming and soccer at the school. He was attending swimming galas which he enjoyed. He began to win medals and this was a great source of joy for us.

Alan received his First Holy Communion and this was a great day for all of us.

His asthma was still monitored by the hospital and he also had his heart and kidneys checked once every two years. His pulmonary stenosis had corrected itself so he did not need surgery. At home we tried to treat Alan as normal. He had to complete household chores which he did not like doing! He was able to set the table or clear it away. Michael worked as a Fitter/Welder and he had a workshop at home. Alan and his brother were always outside with him. They both enjoyed being outdoors.

Every weekend, we went somewhere as a family, visiting places or relations. At this stage Alan was learning how to cycle and was able to kick a football. At night Alan would wander around the house when everyone else was in bed. I am convinced Alan could see in the dark!

At ten years of age he no longer took Locasol; he was eating cheese and any food that you put in front of him and he drank cow's milk. He did not like custard or sauces or ice-cream. He ate a lot of fruit and raw vegetables. He slept well and was busy during the day out and about. He loved to talk to the horses and the birds, he liked the cat. Alan would sit and listen to any type of music.

We became very involved in the Williams Syndrome Association. It was great to attend meetings and hear and speak to other parents about their WS children. We had accepted that Alan had a disability. We were grateful for all that Alan had achieved as we knew other parents who were not as lucky as us.

Our youngest son often asked why Alan was so different to us. We explained that Alan was very sick when he was small and it took him longer to do things. He accepted this and did not ask anymore about it for a year. He was always asking questions and said he wanted a brother like his friends at school. We tried to explain that it was difficult for him to understand what Williams Syndrome was at such a young age but that he would not get it. We would talk to him as he got older and we were learning more about it ourselves also.

Alan himself asked why he was different, why he could not do things that his brother did. We told him that he was very sick for a long time and that it took him longer to do some things but that he was better at swimming than Jason. We also said that everyone is good and bad at different things.

There were many times both of them disagreed as Alan could not tolerate jokes or sarcasm. The solution was to alternate the time spent with either one of us and give them individual attention. It worked well.

When Alan reached eleven years of age he had reached puberty. This caused him some problems—he was increasingly irritable and had pains in his chest. He could not accept the changes. We were told children with Williams Syndrome did not grow very tall, but Alan was growing very fast. We noticed he had a curve on his spine; Alan was referred to an orthopaedic surgeon who said it was very mild but that it should be monitored.

The Williams Syndrome Association was growing steadily by now and we were having weekends away, which we always attended. We met lots of other families and this was a great opportunity to meet and discuss all aspects of Williams Syndrome.

When Alan was twelve he began attending a local disco. He really enjoyed dancing and socialising. This was another great occasion.

Alan's Granddad passed away suddenly in 1992. Alan was very close to him and he could not understand where he had gone to. He used to say goodnight to him every night. Then, in 1999, his Nana died suddenly and Alan asked was anyone else from our family going to Heaven. He was very confused and upset.

Alan was confirmed in 2000. Two weeks after that his father, Michael, died very suddenly. This was a terrible time in our lives and I could not talk to Alan about it. He said that nothing was ever going to be the same again. He did not know how he was going to live. I was unable to talk to him about it or to console him in anyway! I was grieving as well as was his younger brother. He constantly talked about his Dad and things he did with him for years afterwards. This has kept his memory alive. He also wanted to visit the grave. This is not something I want to talk about as I really do not know what to say. My husband's family, my own family, my neighbours and the members of the Williams Syndrome committee were a great source of strength to us during that time.

Alan had counselling and help at school; this seemed to help a little bit. I had become more involved in The Williams Syndrome Association and had taken up the position of Chairperson. In 2001 we had our first Music/Activity camp in Fermanagh. This was well worthwhile for all the campers.

Alan has brought so much joy to us over the years. He is very kind and very much in touch with people's feelings. In 2002, when Alan was sixteen, he was transferred to the adult services at the hospital. Due to his previous calcium problems he was transferred to the endocrinology department where he is seen annually or whenever necessary. His scoliosis did not become any worse but he did have a lot of problems with his knee and hip joints. He was checked by the orthopaedic surgeon and referred for physiotherapy. He had insoles fitted as he had a shortening on one side of his body and this greatly improved his problem. His scoliosis is not causing any problems now.

I noticed Alan was having problems with his eyes again. It seemed like the squint was returning so I brought him to an optician who prescribed glasses. Alan wears glasses all the time now. Alan also had problems with cysts on his upper and lower eyelids. These had to be surgically removed on two occasions and I have been told that this condition can recur.

In 2004 Alan finished his education at the special school. He then began attending a rehabilitative training centre where he has been for the last three years. Alan does not have any problems with his kidneys now. His calcium levels were raised last year so his intake of dairy products has been reduced. His asthma is under control—it is more allergy related—and he takes medication for this once a day. His heart condition is fine—this is monitored every two years—and his blood pressure is good.

In 2005, two of our neighbours died and Alan was badly affected by this. He became very withdrawn, sad and listless, lost weight and, basically, totally changed personality. He was diagnosed with depression and was prescribed medication for this. His GP had to try different medications until he discovered one that suited him.

I think most of this was due to the fact that his father had died when he was thirteen and he had never been able to deal with it properly. He only had counselling for a year and a half consisting of one session every two weeks at our home. His GP tried to reduce his medication but this was unsuccessful. At present he is stabilised with half a tablet daily.

He is in very good form at the moment; the psychologist hopes he will be seen by a Special Needs Psychiatrist to make sure his medication is suiting his needs.

Alan is very involved with the Special Olympics and participated at the national games in basketball last year. He attended the European Youth Games in Rome last year for bocce and he won a silver and a bronze medal. He has numerous swimming medals at both local and regional levels. Alan has also been involved in a local drama group and loves to participate in anything that is going on. He is also learning to play the African drum and enjoys it very much.

Since 2001 Alan has attended the Williams Syndrome Association annual summer camp in Fermanagh. Each year he is maturing and becoming more confident as he enjoys spending time with others as well as playing music. Our Irish WS association is also part of a European WS Federation called FEWS. For the past three years a country from the FEWS group has organised a week long camp. To date this has taken place in Norway, Hungary and Sweden. Alan has attended the camps in both Norway and Sweden. He has no fear of flying and loves getting involved. He even swam in the Artic Ocean while in Norway!

Alan has worked at rehabilitative training for the past three years. This involved computers, art, drama, drums, soccer, cooking, personal and community skills and also work experience. This involves working one half day a week under supervision at Dunne's Stores. He really enjoys this and hopes this is where he will be in the future.

Alan graduated from rehabilitative training in July 2007. Next year he will complete a one year programme called PCP (Person Centred Planning). There he will have a key worker to work with him and our family. He will continue to work in Dunne's Stores for a half day every week.

Alan goes to home sharing once a month where he stays with a family overnight. He attends a disco regularly. Alan also has a volunteer who takes him out to matches, the cinema, and disco or wherever he wishes to go. This allows Alan to become more independent and also gives my other son and myself a break.

Alan has grown into a fine young man. He is very well adjusted and is capable of looking after himself at home and he loves going out. He likes to visit his relations; he is well able to hold a conversation, particularly on sport. Health wise he is doing well. He is six foot in height and has a remarkable memory—he can remember details about people.

He has visited America and France twice, Sweden and Norway. He has also travelled to Cork independently by bus to visit another person with Williams Syndrome. He is still actively involved with the Special Olympics. Alan cannot write very well and has poor reading skills but he is hoping in the next year that he can improve on that. He is a great Liverpool fan and is planning a trip there shortly.

Alan celebrated his 21st birthday party last week. He had a huge party and he really enjoyed it. I never thought I would see the day when Alan would get to that age as he was so sick when he was younger. There have been numerous times over the years when I have cried and been upset because Alan had Williams Syndrome. However, seeing him so happy and seeing what he has achieved has made it all worthwhile. It has made me a better and different person. My other son has been a great support to me over the years especially since Michael died. He intends getting involved with the Williams

Syndrome Association as he gets older. He has great respect for his brother and is very proud of his achievements.

To conclude, I would like to thank everyone who has helped with Alan's upbringing over the years and especially Ann and the Williams Syndrome Association. When I first met Ann I was too busy dealing with all Alan's problems to be as involved as I would have liked to be with the association. Ann always found time to be there, to listen to my issues whenever I contacted her (sometimes late at night!) and I truly appreciate that. Meeting other parents, adult siblings and adult Williams Syndrome people through committee meetings, AGM, weekends away and the music/activity camp has been a tremendous help to me as a mother. Both Alan and Jason have gained lifelong friends through all of those outings and have contact with some of them on a regular basis. They say every mother knows her child best so never give up, as there is someone out there somewhere to help you, that knows what you are going through. I would like to thank Alan for all he has given me over the years. He is witty, sensitive, tall and a charmer with a hearty laugh. He has great courage and has overcome many obstacles in his 21 years.

Alan, all the family are very proud of your achievements and well done. I am looking forward to you maturing and becoming a fine young man who is able to look after himself as the years go by and maybe keep an eye on your Mom too!

The WSAI Story III

SEPTEMBER 1988. I replied to the letter from Galway and life continued on in its own way. My daily routine now invariably involved some work for the WSAI as well as work (both home and away!), taking care of my family and trying to find a little time for myself. Unfortunately, the latter was the thing that generally did not happen!

By this time, I have begun to realise that this work for the association is now taking my money as well as my time! I have been funding all the letter writing, postage, photocopying, etc. out of my own pocket. I decide that the association needs money! I make up a leaflet about the WSAI and I send it with a letter to some companies in the local area. I explain what I am doing and ask for their support. The response I receive is very generous. I am overwhelmed! It is like an affirmation of what we are trying to do. It is like they are saying "I think what you are doing is worthwhile"

The next couple of years roll by. I am, by times, very optimistic for the future of the WSAI and, by times, very pessimistic about it! Towards the end of 1989 I have decided that, if this association is to become something worthwhile, then I will have to be the one to take it on and make it work. I think about this very seriously. This is not the same type of yes/no commitment that has existed for the past couple of years. I realise that the money will have to be raised to further the work. Fundraising did not frighten me but I did not want to embark on it until I had a proper legitimate structure in place.

And so the process of getting the WSAI registered as a charity started. I spoke to many people and received many helpful suggestions. I contacted the Revenue Commissioners to find out what was required and they said I needed a constitution. So I drafted a constitution and presented this at a meeting for discussion. After a number of meetings a final wording was agreed between the WS families. I sent this with a letter of application to the Revenue Commissioners on 11 September 1989.

I thought the charity registration would take a couple of months!! How wrong I was! There were a number of adjustments to the constitution required by the Revenue so communications passed to and fro for some time. Finally, on 5 November 1991 (2 years later!), I received official notification of the association's registration as a charitable organisation.

During this time, new WS families continued to contact me. One of these contacts was from Robert's family during September 1989. The story was again very similar to Alan's story but Robert, at this time, was in his mid 20's. His family had been in touch with the IHC in the UK in earlier years.

Making contact with this family was very important to the other members of the WSAI, mainly because of Robert's age. We felt that we could learn so much about what the future held for our WS youngsters by talking to them. And we did! The family was very open and helpful. They answered all the questions posed to them as well as they could. I will always be extremely grateful to them for the friendship and support they showed to me and to all the members of the WSAI.

Robert's Story

WHEN I WAS FIRST ASKED TO WRITE an article on my son, I thought, OK. His and our experiences might be of some encouragement to those who have had a child diagnosed with WS.

I started to write, rewrite, but couldn't go any further than his childhood years. I felt I was invading his privacy, as he is now forty years old.

So I am trying once again having been encouraged to do so.

Robert was our first-born, arriving three weeks later than expected. Weight 7lbs 10ozs. He went straight into an incubator, was put on a subcutaneous drip for dehydration and pyrexia. (A chance glance at a radiologist's report years later suggested he had pneumonia. Didn't believe it then, still don't!) He would still be in the incubator if his dad hadn't demanded he be brought down to be fed by his mother!

The first thing I noticed—besides being gorgeous—was that he cried a lot before and after feeds and vomited. Being a midwife, I knew this was not the norm. The midwife observed "Well, you of all people should know, he's only regurgitating." Only regurgitating! At six days, he came home and he cried, fed, vomited, slept for long periods, had severe constipation and gained a couple of ounces a week, if lucky. I had to give up feeding him myself as I couldn't keep up with his demands as he vomited so often. But he was even worse on cow's milk. Still, we persevered. We had to, as our own doctor would remark "Are you starving him or what?"

The crunch came when Robert was about eight months old. I lifted him from his cot and out of a pool of urine. I couldn't believe the amount from such a tiny mite—now 15 lbs. I had him admitted to a particular Nursing Home outside Cork where I had previously nursed and where I knew he would get A1 treatment. Quite honestly I didn't expect him to come home again. He was so ill and listless.

However, five weeks later, we brought him home with strict instructions as regards diet. It had been noticed by the staff also, that he vomited when given certain foods but, in particular, milk and milky foods. Advice given: give half strength milk and gradually increase to full strength. We did that but ended up back at square one again. He was also prescribed iron drops and Abidec. But he wasn't given then immediately because I didn't know what we were treating.

At 11 months, the next step was to a professor of paediatrics. Having got Robert's history he suggested the problem might be oesophageal reflux or hiatus hernia. He advised us to sit him up for six weeks, day and night. So dad made a wooden armchair-type upright seat and padded it. Still no change in Robert's condition

Back to the professor. He suggested several diagnoses but then abandoned them. Finally, a blood sample was sent to the North of Ireland for analysis. Result: calcium content extremely high. He reckoned there had been a mistake so asked for another test. Result: even higher calcium content. So we had a diagnosis—Idiopathic Infantile Hypercalcaemia. Sounded very impressive! Nowadays it is, of course, Williams Syndrome.

And so, at 13 months, Robert started on Locasol (milk replacement) and from that day to this he has seldom vomited.

If anyone in his company is liable to throw up, he's gone! His grandfather described Locasol as "the ground-up bones of the previous victim!" It wasn't very pleasant but it did the trick. It was also very expensive.

He had such a poor start that he was quite feeble and his muscle tone was very weak.

The arrival of his sister when Robert was 16 months was a blessing. It meant I had to share myself between the two and not concentrate totally on one. It was like having twins and, although it was hard work, she was a tonic in disguise!

We had noticed that Robert didn't like noise (hyperacusis). The vacuum cleaner, a noisy truck passing his pram, dad hammering or using an electric drill, all affected him. But then, other children object to these types of noises too. To us, he was just hypersensitive. But, oh boys, it was when his sister cried that we realised that noise played a part in his problem.

It must be remembered that little or nothing at all, was known about Williams Syndrome by doctors or paediatricians (except our prof.) in Ireland at that time.

Feeding was always a problem. He was allowed apples and bananas. The latter couldn't be bought all year round at that time but, from time to time, we were given a box as they arrived in port. They had to be imported green so they lasted for some time in the fridge. It helped to know the right people! Before flour was used by bakers, certain supplements were added. Mills were not allowed, by law, to sell it in its original state. So all "floury" foods were out. Margarine was recommended as opposed to butter. But, as I pointed out, the wrapper stated that vitamins A and D were added to the margarine.

So back to butter! Robert took an instant dislike to anything that had previously made him vomit so it was some time before he sorted himself out on a diet that suited him and that he liked.

Knowing this, his sister, even at 18 months, teased him unmercifully with food (like rusks) she knew he wasn't allowed to have. So she had to be watched. Nowadays, Robert eats a normal diet.

Another major problem: he wasn't allowed out in the sun because of the vitamin D factor which is essential for the absorption of calcium. Dad made a large three-sided and roofed tent in which Robert could play or rest. Any outings were made in the evenings.

From an early age he took to machines. Anything with bolts, screws, wires or knobs. He took them to pieces; we cleared them up. His dad brought home engines and even made up Meccano for him to take apart. He took my old washing machine apart! (May 2003)! However, at a later age he spent every Saturday with a family of hauliers and became very knowledgeable about truck engines.

At 21 years of age, he was given a C.B. radio and coped with it brilliantly. I was the "doubting Thomas" but dad was confident he could cope with it. He got to know and meet truckers. He would chat on and on and on.... until they were out of radio range. For the last fifteen years he has many times accompanied a trucker to the continent delivering goods. A great way to see the world!

But I have jumped ahead.

At 2 years old, I noticed a slight squint in Robert's left eye. I took him to see an optician. Result: very long sighted. He would have to wear glasses constantly. He was under regular supervision. It was hoped that exercises and covering one lens from time to time would correct the lazy eye but, finally, at 8 years of age the squint was surgically corrected.

As Robert's height and weight were below average and a concern to the professor's team, he underwent a series of very unpleasant tests for growth hormones. Results: they said he would probably grow another six inches, which was very encouraging. The cost of the hormone treatment would have run into thousands of pounds over a six or seven year treatment period. He had several prescribed periods of thyroxine during the time everyone was worried about his development. He went through measles, mumps, chicken pox and German measles. He suffered from severe hay fever each spring/summer. He was banished, to his delight, to his grandparents when we had glandular fever in the house.

Like most WS children, he had a preference for the company of older children or adults rather than children of his own age. He could always stand up and give a speech, quite unabashed and with great aplomb!

He attended the dentist from an early age, every six months regularly to the present day and more often if necessary. His last milk tooth came out when he was 19 years old. He has had teeth extracted to make room for others, which have become impacted in the gum or decided to appear in the palate of the mouth. His teeth are very irregular and certainly need constant care.

At five and a half years he started primary school with his sister. He found it difficult but liked the company. Writing was very laborious as his eye coordination was poor. In 6th class it was obvious that he was holding back the class although the teacher did what she could. So we decided to have him assessed by a psychologist. Result: he started in what is now called COPE at 12 years of age. He gained a very good grounding in writing, reading and simple sums.

At 15 he started in VTC where he got a taste of various workshops. He hated, and was scared stiff of, the speed and noise of the wood lathe. He enjoyed the printing room but there was no future there for him.

He went through a stage of being bullied. Being short in stature, he was an easy target for the bigger boys. I found out that he was eating his lunch on his way to school so that it wouldn't be taken from him later in the day. He was also pushed about at the bus stop on the way home. Once I found out, I reported it and it was dealt with well and efficiently.

At 19 he got a place in Cork Regional Hospital, renamed

Cork University Hospital. After a trial period he was made permanent. It was referred to as sheltered employment. He was trained to fix wheels and, when you think about it, there are many wheels in a hospital!

At 20 Robert complained of a pain in his back. He was given medication that relieved it for a while. Eventually, however, he was diagnosed as having scoliosis of the spine. The orthopaedic specialist maintained that he had had it for about nine years but it had only become evident when he started work at 19. Result: no surgical treatment. The scoliosis was too developed. Painkillers, and rest whenever required, were prescribed.

He had several bouts of cystitis and over time had a series of tests: cystoscopy, ultrasound, cystogram and IVP and numerous consultations with urologists. His bladder is small with several diverticula. These compensate for the size of the bladder and, if they were removed, Robert would be passing urine every half hour or so. On X-ray his bladder looks like a sea mine! But if it works, leave well alone.

He had two bouts of retention of urine following the death of his dad. This could be due to a psychological factor—my diagnosis—as no other cause was found after having spent two weeks in hospital each time.

In 1996, Robert suddenly experienced very severe abdominal pain. I reckoned it wasn't appendicitis but after a couple of hours when his temperature and pulse rose, he was admitted to Cork University Hospital and kept under observation all night. Nothing showed on X-ray. He was taken to theatre for a laparotomy that resulted in a colostomy. An infected diverticulum had burst in the colon. He dealt with it quite well on the whole but it wasn't nice, as he says himself. Fortunately, seven months later, it was reversed satisfactorily.

After some months Robert developed gynaecomastia (enlarged breast) and last year had a mastectomy.

He is, once again, experiencing abdominal discomfort

in the area of the previous operations and is attending the appropriate clinic.

One wonders—what next?

In 2002 Robert received his 20 year Service Pin and Scroll in Cork University Hospital. The staff in the canteen made him a cake in the shape of a truck with all its appropriate bits. He was thrilled with all this, as you can imagine! His dad would have been so proud of him as indeed are his two brothers and his sister. And, of course, me, his mum!

Robert was 40 years old in May 2003 and my birthday present to him was a holiday with the entire family—brothers, sister, brother-in-law, two sisters-in-law, two nieces and three nephews. He had a wonderful time!!

The WSAI Story IV

1990. I AM IN CONTACT WITH Professor Bryan Hall. He will be travelling to England in September/October this year to attend a medical conference. I ask him to stop off in Ireland and give a talk at a meeting that I will organise. He is, as always, obliging and arrives in Ireland in September. I hold the meeting in Ballinasloe on Thursday 27th September. There is quite a good turnout at the meeting—both WS family members and medical people. During his talk that evening, I hear the first mention of the cause of Williams Syndrome. Bryan tells us that genetic research at that point has determined that the cause of WS is based in Chromosome No 7. He says that they need better technology and further research to be able to determine the exact cause.

In 1993, I read that the cause of WS is missing genetic material (particularly the gene that governs elastin) in Chromosome No. 7. Bryan was right, almost three years earlier!

November 1991. Registered Charity No. 9654! I will have to get new letter headed paper!

How many member families do we have now? Not many still! Still hard to get people to meetings so I decide to start sending out a "newsletter." It is using the term "newsletter" very lightly really! It is just a couple of pages of information to try to keep in touch with all the member families. I am continuing to get contact from a new family now and then, so I think it is very important to try to maintain contact and to enlarge the family circle.

One new family that contacts me in November 1991 is Adrienne's family. Adrienne is now almost 16 years of age and, again, we are all very anxious to meet her and talk to her parents. Their experience will be invaluable to us. And so it is!

Over the following years many families get in touch with the WSAI looking for help and support. We do our best to supply this help and support. Some of the stories of these families are told in the following pages.

Adrienne's Story

ADRIENNE WAS BORN IN DEC 1975. She was a full term baby, the birth was normal and she weighed 6lbs 2ozs. This weight was considerably less than any of our three previous children who each weighed approximately 10lbs. In the weeks following her birth the only defect we noticed was that both of her eyes were quite badly turned in. We jokingly called them suspicious eyes, as they seemed to watch each other. One eye was corrected at Our Lady's Children's Hospital Dublin when Adrienne was 2 years of age.

At the beginning Adrienne appeared to be a little slow. She was very slow to feed compared to our other children. During a visit by the local clinic nurse she suggested, as Adrienne seemed to be making poor progress, that we should have her checked out at Our Lady's Hospital. A report received after this check confirmed that Adrienne was acting slow for her age but otherwise was quite healthy. It was recommended that we treat Adrienne as we had our other children and to enjoy her.

From the age of 2 to 5 years Adrienne had a problem which caused us considerable upset. She would have severe tummy upsets each week lasting for at least four days at a time. Our GP at the time was a young man we found quite unhelpful.

On one occasion, when we insisted on some action by him he gave a letter to arrange a Barium Meal test that stated we were just very fussy parents. The test, when completed, did not indicate the cause of the vomiting nor did it help with any diagnosis. The problem persisted and we continued to deal with it as best we could.

At 7 years of age Adrienne had her second eye corrected and has used glasses since. During this procedure, concern was expressed over a possible heart defect, which showed up at the time. A Dr. Duff, Our Lady's Children's Hospital then became involved and it was only at this time, after seeing her, that her features identified to him that she was a Williams Syndrome baby. Dr. Duff provided leaflets explaining the condition that affected Adrienne and we were very glad to have Adrienne's condition at last identified. We were told that Williams Syndrome was worldwide but that very few medical practitioners had any experience of it or could identify it although, as parents, it is quite apparent to us when we see children with it.

At that time it was also confirmed that Adrienne had mitral valve prolapse and regurgitation, hence her ongoing tummy upsets. From this time Adrienne has had to have regular heart and eye tests and at 21 years of age she was transferred to the Mater Hospital where she has annual checks. A very recent heart check confirmed a big improvement in her heart valves so her next appointment is in two years.

At the tender age of 2 and a half years Adrienne started attending a local Montessori school. There she mixed in very well with the other children. However, it was also clearly identified that Adrienne was indeed very slow. Adrienne was always in good humour and very easy to please. She stayed in the Montessori school until 5 and a half years of age when we were very fortunate to find a suitable primary school for her. This was the Special Unit, St. Ann's, Milltown, Dublin which also had a secondary school.

Until Adrienne was twelve she was collected each morning and brought to St. Ann's in a mini bus along with other children picked up along the way and each afternoon was delivered safely home. With her constant smile and good humour Adrienne easily won the hearts of the lady driver, the schoolteachers who were excellent and all of the pupils in her class. She would give you a smile and a hug when leaving for school and the same again on her return. When she came home she always had to have a half an hour with her Mom—this continues to this day—to explain all that has happened while she was away and, of course, wanting to know what happened during our day.

At 9 years of age Adrienne had her first period. This was very traumatic for her. However, it was explained in full detail to her by her Mom and accepted as a minor hurdle in life.

In St. Ann's we were very fortunate that they had a small swimming pool where they provided instruction for their pupils. Within a very short time Adrienne became very comfortable in the water and progressed from using armbands to swimming in a very short time. We were very pleased with this, as all of our family are quite competent swimmers and always enjoyed seaside holidays.

At 12 years of age Adrienne progressed through to the secondary special unit in St. Ann's and her collection and delivery to school by minibus ceased. This posed problems for us as to get there by public transport required taking two buses with the changeover taking place in Ranelagh Village, a very busy area. To deal with this, during the summer holidays we started taking the bus to St. Ann's until we thought Adrienne would know her way. At all times we fully explained what we were doing and what we would expect of her. Finally we decided to put her to the test, putting her on the bus and letting her make her own way to school. Unaware that we followed her in a car she did as she had practiced and arrived safe and sound and, of course, delighted to find us waiting for her. In this way Adrienne made her way home every school day.

In the morning she was brought by car and during our journey we used the time to play various games. As Adrienne was now reading we held 'Spelling Bees' and her competence at this was very pleasing. We also did 'Maths Tables,' subtraction, addition etc., which always shortened our journeys. She enjoyed best our games with car registration numbers. This required her to know all of our counties and identifying each and every car to its county of registration. In a short time she could tell every county by a registration plate. To develop her concentration we developed many similar games that kept us busy and helped her.

At this time at home we became involved in the Community Games and, along with another family, founded our own swimming club. Through our efforts Adrienne's swimming improved greatly and we were quite satisfied with her progress and competence. Through her school we were asked to allow Adrienne represent St. Ann's at a forthcoming gala arranged for children with disabilities. Adrienne was quite small at 13 years and at the gala we were aghast to see the size of most of the other competitors. Most of them were at least 12 inches taller than her. We needn't have worried.

Through the heats and finals for her age she proved she was the best and brought home two gold medals. As she was the only competitor from her school the organisers were very surprised and indeed when she brought her medals to show to her friends and teachers they were so proud of her. Adrienne represented her school for four years altogether and although the competition got harder as she grew older she always came home with at least a gold and silver medal. A lot of our time was spent helping to improve Adrienne's ability in every activity and we are pleased and proud of her successes. It was well worth the effort.

Another activity we practiced was cycling. At first we bought Adrienne a tricycle and as she grew we would get her a bigger bike until we ended up with a juvenile bike fitted with stabilisers. From the beginning Adrienne was not very happy, as she seemed to have a slight balance problem. When going up a stairs Adrienne would always make sure that her full foot was on the step before she would move to the next one. In the mid eighties it was quite safe to cycle around Dublin roads. There were relatively few cars on the road but there were plenty of cyclists.

To get Adrienne used to her new bicycle and stabilisers we would take her, on each fine Sunday morning, to St. Stephen's Green. At that time there were no problems with parking and traffic went each way around The Green. People who know Dublin will know that the pavement around The Green is very wide—it is as wide as a roadway in any housing estate—and at 10am on a Sunday morning there are few or no pedestrians. For about 2 hours we would practice cycling around The Green and, as her skills improved, the stabilisers' assistance was reduced until we eventually removed them altogether. This was when my problems started.

In the beginning, because Adrienne cycled quite slowly, there was no difficulty in keeping up with her but as she improved so also did her speed. Eventually I had to use my own bike to stay close to her and can honestly say her progress was a delight to all of our family. And she still smiled and stayed in good humour.

Because of her success around The Green, we then went to practice on the cycle track in Sandrive Park. This is a banked cycle bowl that was difficult to manage at first but again progress was inevitable. We did this for some time and then decided on a major change. Adrienne was quite relaxed on her cycle and was quite strong so we decided to do some road work. Again, one has to remember that in the eighties it was quite safe to ride on the road and there was only a fraction of present day traffic on the road then.

What we arranged to do was, again on each fine Sunday morning, starting at 10am, to cycle up the Grand Canal to Inchicore, then out the Naas Road to the Long Mile Road and return home, a distance of at least seven miles. We did this trip for some months and then, taking the same route and using the hard shoulder, went on to Newlands Cross, returning home through Tallaght, again a distance of about 10 miles. Things went so well that we again decided to lengthen our spin.

We went the usual way as far as Newlands Cross. Then we continued along the Naas Road as far as Saggart Village where we stopped for a picnic and ice cream before returning home through Tallaght, a distance of up to 17 miles. Even in the biggest area the hills were no problem to Adrienne who still continued to be a good humoured and happy person.

We continued this particular spin for some months and only stopped when winter came. In this particular exercise we, the parents, had to work very hard at it but the results were immensely rewarding. In hindsight, we worked all the time on Adrienne's strengths i.e. swimming, cycling and the games going to school in the car. They were all of immense benefit to Adrienne and each success was a gain for each and every member of our family. We, of course, worked on her weaknesses and our efforts and those of her teachers, friends and, latterly, her colleagues at work have produced a very good humoured, caring and capable daughter. It was very hard work at times but the end result is the satisfaction of her company.

While in St. Ann's, a female officer from the National Rehabilitation Board (NRB) was responsible for keeping a check on all of the children there with 'Special Needs.' We were never pleased with this service, as this officer did not seem to place any importance on the development of these children. The attention given by the teachers and principal was marvellous. It was indeed a very happy school.

Towards the end of Adrienne's schooling we expected to have a meeting with the NRB and to discuss with them the options we would have for Adrienne. It was only when we made contact with them that we were told it was now our responsibility to decide what path should follow for her future. We felt their attitude to say the least was unhelpful as they were supposed to be the experts in these matters and should have been able to assist and advise us on at least what was available.

At all times during Adrienne's life we could never go to a government department and be told what was available for children with disabilities. Instead we always had to do our own investigations and when we had our information and presented it to a department it was always amazing how quickly the relevant information would be provided. We always had to do the donkeywork, which in turn was passed on to our WS Association after it was founded by Ann Breen some years ago.

Through our own efforts we discovered a list of training centres for people with 'special needs.' We phoned each and made appointments to see the centres, to check what activities were carried out in each and also how it would suit Adrienne. We were very impressed with the Rehab Centre (now NDTI) in Broomhill Road, Tallaght. The management and staff whom we interviewed came across as very caring and genuine people and, after discussions with Adrienne, we placed her name on their waiting list. After a short period a vacancy occurred so Adrienne, at 19 years of age, became a trainee with Rehab. For the first year she did their academic course where she was frequently assessed.

She did a number of 'assertiveness' courses which became second nature to her and her confidence improved immensely. Now she will stand her ground and argue her case with anyone. We also insisted that Adrienne speak her mind and not be afraid of expressing her opinion. She doesn't like loud arguments and will always try to pour oil on troubled waters. She is very caring and will always remember people's hurts, injuries or illnesses and, although months may pass before they meet again, she will always ask about their past problems.

Adrienne trained in electronics with Rehab for three years and was very happy there. She became an 'agony' aunt for most of her friends there who would discuss most of their problems with her.

Then one day she heard that a local supermarket was willing to provide work experience for a few trainees. Adrienne jumped at the chance, it was a new challenge for her and the supermarket was only six or seven minutes walk from home. She was accepted and worked there for six weeks. She was delighted with the busy atmosphere and was very contented with the supervisors and staff.

At the end of the six weeks she went to the manager and told him that she wanted a job there. She told him that she would work very hard, that the customers all spoke highly of her to the supervisors and that he would be missing out on an excellent worker if he didn't offer her a job. As he had seen her work for six weeks and was satisfied that she could do as she had said, he offered her a job saying she had sold herself to him. We were delighted to hear what Adrienne had done. She was delighted as she now had a job and she was earning a wage.

We would describe Adrienne as a 'people person.' She is very happy particularly in older people's company but is also happy with younger children.

On every occasion, Adrienne is a joy to be with although she doesn't have a great sense of humour and is perhaps inclined to be a little too serious. Her sister and brothers are amazed at, and indeed very proud of, her achievements and give support to her as required.

Superquinn is the name of the supermarket where Adrienne works. They are an excellent employer and have a policy of providing employment to those with disabilities. By agreement with management Adrienne works three mornings per week, to stay within the constraints of the DA benefit. Any extra hours worked would affect her allowances.

For the remaining two mornings each week Adrienne attends Crumlin Road College for English, Maths and Computers. She expects to receive a certificate in June for each subject. Again with her smile and humour she has an excellent relationship with both teachers and students there.

Adrienne swims twice a week, walks at least twenty miles,

mainly with her Mom who is like her bigger sister, but doesn't cycle. She helps out in our church by being a collector and is always very pleased when she has done more work than any other collector. She loves eating out and is happiest when we go away to the sun. She is very good with money, has a weakness for jewellery and loves her music. On completing a walk she never fails to say 'Yes. I enjoyed the walk.' Some months ago we read an article on Williams Syndrome which concluded— if you should have to have a child with a disability than you would be blessed if you had one with Williams Syndrome which could have been called the 'Happy Syndrome.'

In our experience this would be a very accurate description of Adrienne who, over the years, has provided us with countless hours of good humour, pleasure and happy memories. We have faced many difficult moments but when you see the welcoming face looking and smiling at you the difficulties diminish and your efforts are rewarded.

Through leaflets provided by Dr. Duff we heard of the foundation of 'The Williams Syndrome Association of Ireland' quite some years ago. We made contact with the founder, Ann Breen, joined the association and became committee members. We have been involved in various activities to raise the profile of our association, have fund raised and have spoken to doctors on our association.

Because Adrienne is one of our older 'Williams' children on weekends away we have been able to talk to newer members on many of the problems they are likely to face, what entitlements they have and the best means of dealing with specific difficulties. We are making slow progress but like the snail we will get there in the end. We are indebted to Ann Breen for all her efforts and we wish to thank her and her committee for their tremendous efforts.

To all the parents of WS children we say—it is a fact of life that, through their good humour, WS children make friends very easily but it is also a sad fact that they also lose them easily. Because the average child develops into our ever-changing world at a faster rate than a WS child, they lose contact with each other and eventually separate going their own ways while still remaining friendly to each other.

In the past Adrienne, when she realised that she was somewhat different to many of her friends, would ask some awkward and searching questions. We never avoided these questions always answering them in an honest and full way. From an early age we discussed items of household interest with her and, in later years, included her in every decision that we made. We would discuss items of expenditure with her. When decorating, we would get her views on colours and involve her in every way so that she could understand the cost of running a home. We have endeavoured to get her honest opinion on almost everything we are about to do and we honestly try to treat her as an equal.

Of major concern to us is what is to happen to Adrienne when we pass on. We have our other children who, no doubt, will help to take care of her. However, there is an age difference of 10 and 20 years between them and Adrienne. They are all married and there is every reason to suppose that certain difficulties could arise between their spouses and children and therefore it would not be right to impose changes into their lives and habits.

As there are no records of life expectancy with WS people, we have to assume that most WS people will enjoy a full and long life. In our case, Adrienne could quite easily survive her sister and brothers. In this regard, we cannot, at this time, make full plans for this eventuality and therefore can only leave this in the hands of God.

Patricia's Story

PATRICIA WAS DIAGNOSED WITH WS when she was 5 years old, though of course we knew much earlier that she wasn't quite 'normal.' We had gone through the poor feeding, colic, sleepless nights, developmental delays and quirks that are typical of Williams. In comparison to others we've spoken with or read about, though, we had a relatively easy ride. Once she was diagnosed she was checked regularly for the various physical problems associated with WS, but again nothing serious manifested itself.

From our point of view, therefore, the major impact of WS has been the learning disability, and also the poor motor skills, and we have had several decisions to make regarding her education over the years.

Patricia was so sociable from an early age that we started her in a playgroup when she was only 2, before we knew anything about her WS. Shortly after this she had her first psychological assessment (because of her developmental delays). Her psychologist was a bit baffled by her uneven development but, the bottom line was, she was about a year delayed. I was devastated by this news—she was our first child and I didn't really have any experience of children, none of my friends or colleagues had children, she was the first grandchild in my family, so I had no comparison to measure her by.

In subsequent assessments this delay varied slightly, sometimes improving, sometimes falling back again, and the psychologist did her best to reassure me that if Patricia maintained that same gap consistently, then the older she got the less it would matter. She did point out, however, that she might eventually reach a plateau in her development beyond which she couldn't go.

When Patricia's playgroup closed (shortly after that first assessment) she started in a new one that was very Montessori-based. She absolutely adored this group, cried when she had to go home (I used to worry people would think I mistreated her at home!), so when we moved house when Patricia was just 4 I chose a local Montessori school for her.

My policy by now was to treat Patricia as if she was a year younger than she actually was and I hoped to be able to send her to the local girls' National School when she was 6. This Montessori school was not a playgroup, but a school that followed the Montessori method very fully, and it soon became apparent that Patricia was exhibiting learning difficulties and had great difficulty learning to write.

Advice was sought from her psychologist concerning schooling and her recommendation was to leave Patricia in this school which, it transpired, had a great reputation for dealing with children with learning disability. It also had a senior class for children from 6–9 years old and would therefore be ideal for Patricia, as the psychologist felt she was too distractible to cope with mainstream schooling.

So, for six years, Patricia attended this Montessori school. It had its benefits and its problems. The Montessori teaching method suited Patricia, particularly the phonic-based reading method, and the discipline and routine were very good for her. The small class size was ideal. However, I often felt that, in the junior class at least, there was insufficient reward in the form of stars or even praise when something was achieved, while there seemed to be plenty of criticism when it wasn't. I tackled the teacher about this and her reply was that the achievement was reward in itself. She didn't seem to take on board that, for Patricia, this was not the case and a little bit of praise (or even a lot of it!) could have worked wonders. I'm not sure to this day if this was really the Montessori method or just this particular teacher being too rigid. It got to the point where Patricia didn't like her teacher, didn't want to go to school, and her last year in the junior class was very difficult. However, we stuck it out because we knew that the senior class would be better and, frankly, we didn't know of any alternative.

It was while Patricia was in the junior class in her Montessori school that we got the WS diagnosis. I think it was at this point that I started to wonder if Patricia should be in special schooling but I was concerned that, if she were, she would copy any and every behaviour and bad habit she encountered because she was so imitative.

In discussions with the psychologist, the conclusion again was to leave her in the Montessori school for now. The psychologist felt that Patricia was too little and physically vulnerable for our nearest Special School, where the children are mostly very able-bodied, but that it would probably be an option later.

The senior Montessori class was quite good for Patricia. She blossomed quite a bit during those three years. Her reading, in particular, took off and her confidence returned. She made her First Communion and read the Responsorial Psalm perfectly at the ceremony. I formulated a plan for her education up to 18! I would keep her at the Montessori school till she was 11 going on 12 (this had been done with others) and she was accepted in the special class of a girl's secondary school for when she was 12. Unfortunately, none of this worked out!

The secondary school closed, and then the numbers in the senior Montessori class dropped so low that they were forced to close also! Her third year there would have to be her last. She would be going on 10 when she finished there.

In a panic most of the mothers of the children in Patricia's class started looking for alternatives. In a class of eight children, six had a learning disability of some sort, ranging from dyslexia to a few genetic disorders. We mothers had, over the years, forged very good friendships, had supported each other through various difficulties concerning our children and most of us are still in regular contact. We now went, almost en-masse, to the various alternative schools, and, in the end, for Patricia it came down to a choice between the previously mentioned Special School and a reasonably close (but not local) mainstream National School with a well-spoken of Special Unit which catered for a wider catchment area.

She was readily accepted at both schools following assessments, and we opted for the mainstream school for a number of reasons. Firstly, the organisation of the Special Unit would not be too different from the Montessori school, with small classes and a mix of age and ability. Secondly, the teacher in what would be Patricia's class (the senior of the Unit's 3 classes) was Montessori trained. And finally, the staff we met—the Acting Principal, the Special Unit Head and the Senior Class Teacher—were wonderful. The Special School was still the most likely option for later.

Patricia's first year in the Special Unit didn't go as well as we had hoped! Again, for a number of reasons. None of the staff we had met were actually in the Unit. The Montessori-trained Class Teacher didn't have her appointment sanctioned by the Department of Education (who seem to have a problem with Montessori training), the Unit Head was away on a Special Education training course which, in the long run, would benefit the Unit but for that year left it floundering a bit and the Acting Principal retired! Patricia and a boy in her class developed a profound antagonism for one another that made discipline very difficult for their lovely but inexperienced teacher and puberty kicked in for Patricia.

Academically, Patricia's writing and maths were problematic. Her teacher was surprised at just how weak her maths was, despite having read all the literature on WS that I provided. That first year was extremely difficult. Patricia was obviously unhappy and I wondered had I made a major mistake in sending her there, until I started to hear similar stories concerning the Special School from the mother of one of Patricia's former classmates.

We struggled through the year and by her second year things started to settle down. Patricia was moved between the different classes in the Special Unit according to her ability, going to the junior class for maths, and this seemed to suit her. The Head of the Unit was back from her training course and provided a stabilising influence. She was coping better with her antagonistic classmate. Patricia was integrated with mainstream classes for music and choir and took part in the Hallelujah Concert as part of a 2,000-strong children's choir in the Point Depot. She was happier.

Half way through her second year, the Unit Head contacted me concerning where Patricia would go next. She said that if I planned on sending Patricia to the Special School, then she would need to go the following September as she would then be old enough to leave National School. However, if I wanted to send Patricia to mainstream Secondary School, then the Department of Education could be persuaded to leave her an extra year in National School on the grounds that, because of her learning disability, she would benefit from the extra year. I was stunned for two reasons.

Firstly, I had no intention of moving Patricia to the Special School so soon—she was only just settling down where she was. I had assumed she would be there for three years. To move her again was unthinkable! Secondly, I hadn't considered mainstream Secondary School as an option. The Unit Head felt that, with the extra year, Patricia would be perfectly capable of attending mainstream Secondary School provided she had the appropriate Learning Support. She suggested visiting Secondary Schools in my area to see if one was suitable.

I did this and was pleasantly surprised to discover that the three schools I visited would all be quite happy to take Patricia as a student. One of these schools (a Community School) was well ahead of the others in terms of providing the appropriate support so the choice was easy.

Patricia did her third year in the Special Unit, blossoming once again in confidence and ability, and then started Secondary School with a full-time Special Needs Assistant, a lovely lady who takes no nonsense from Patricia. The school keeps one class each year small (about 15 students) for weaker students, and this is the class she is placed in. The school Resource Teacher is her class tutor, and he also takes the class for English and is the Remedial Teacher sitting in during Maths classes.

Maths is now one of her best subjects! She is doing this at foundation level and can cope quite well with the help of her calculator. Her English teacher says she is one of the strongest in the class (also foundation level) in terms of language ability and comprehension. She is now just finished Second Year, does a full range of core and optional subjects, but is exempt from Irish (does Resource work during this class). Her handwriting is the only major problem but the Resource Teacher is hoping to arrange a scribe and/or dictating answers into a tape recorder for her Junior Cert. Yes, they are actually saying she can pass her Junior Cert!

But the most important thing is that Patricia is very happy at this school even though she grumbles about the homework.

Brian's Story

BRIAN WAS BORN ON THE 8TH NOVEMBER 1967, a small baby 6lbs 7oz. For his first 6 months he was in and out of hospital, first with acute pneumonia that led to an inguinal hernia that led to gastroenteritis. During this stay in hospital Brian was diagnosed with hypercalcaemia, which resulted in soft bones and slow development. Williams syndrome was never mentioned. It was some years before we discovered he had WS.

Through diet, Brian's calcium levels were brought under control and, from then on, he began to make progress, though somewhat slower than usual. He was assessed on a yearly basis and at around 5 years was sent to primary school and settled in well, due to his outgoing and very friendly personality. In common with all WS children Brian displayed a fear of loud noises and a liking for the wind but, as an adult, is no longer affected to any great extent.

From about second class onwards Brian cycled to school every day, a journey of about 2 miles and he knew everyone on the route. After primary school, he studied at the local secondary school and continued on to sit his intermediate certificate exam. He was successful in passing a number of subjects, including History, English, French and Geography. Maths was something else!

After his intermediate certificate exam, Brian left school and went to FAS to do a three-month youth project, followed by a 6-week metal work course. He then went to work in REHAB and stayed with them for almost 10 years.

He left REHAB to pursue a music course in Dublin, living there for nearly two years. He was successful and was awarded an NTDI certificate for music, sound engineering, piano, communication, process studies and the music industry. During this time Brian was a stage manager for a concert in Temple Bar music centre and also travelled to Denmark and Germany, working with other groups preparing and producing musical plays.

Back in Cork, Brian spent 9 months in the APW factory, working on the assembly line. Here he made disk drives and after that went to work in FAS as a general assistant. He has been made a permanent member of the staff in FAS and this is where he is currently employed.

Brian's interest in music started at a very early age. He was always to be found playing away at the piano keys. If he was feeling unsure or sad he found comfort playing the piano. He was sent to music lessons but displayed little interest. However, in his own time he became very proficient and at every party in the house Brian was, and is, our musical entertainer. Down through the years he has played for parties and functions, friends and relatives, clubs and pubs. This year he composed a piece of music for his sister to celebrate her marriage and now, due to great demand, is recording it.

Motorbikes are Brian's other great interest and he has been riding bikes for many years. He is presently driving a Suzuki 250, but would very much like a Harley Davidson! He is a member of Shamrock Rovers MCC and can be regularly found travelling around the countryside on his motorbike with his friends on charity runs.

Conor's Story

CONOR WAS BORN ON 13/12/2000 BY caesarean section and two weeks overdue. He spent the first days of his life in the special care unit in Our Lady's Hospital, Drogheda. It was here that they picked up on Conor's heart murmur but we were told that it was not very significant and that in time it might disappear altogether.

I took him home to Navan exactly 7 days later and we were more or less given the all clear with him. We were not to know then but our life as we knew it was over and a whole new chapter was about to begin which was to be filled with all kinds of feelings and emotions.

What followed in the next six to eight months was definitely the hardest and most difficult challenge I have ever faced in my life to date.

Conor was a very irritable and sick baby. He cried almost non-stop and vomited everything that we struggled so hard to get into him. His sleeping pattern was so bad he only ever slept for short periods before he woke screaming. He was a really bad feeder and I spent most of the day trying to get him to take his bottle. We have one other daughter who was just over 2 yrs when Conor was born. I just found trying to cope with Conor being so sick and difficult and trying to give Aoife attention as well was very hard. The sleep deprivation was really getting to me.

I would say that Conor was about 4 weeks old when I started to have suspicions that something was just not right with him. He was so unresponsive and never seemed to have any kind of reaction by way of a smile or a gesture that you would have expected at that stage. His face had such a blank look on it all the time. I used to look at his face and think that his eyes were very far apart and that he was very unusual looking.

As time went on it was becoming obvious that Conor's development was somewhat delayed. At 12 weeks Conor was admitted to Our Lady's Hospital for Sick Children in Crumlin with chronic projectile vomiting. He had wasted away to almost nothing and was so underweight that he had become almost emaciated. We were so worried about him at this stage and he was so ill. They eventually did a pyloric stenosis operation.

This was to remove a blockage from his stomach that was causing all the vomiting. This procedure has a 100% success rate but, in Conor's case, just 6 weeks later he was still as bad as ever, just projectile vomiting everything that he swallowed. We were at the end of our tether. I was so exhausted as was my husband Martin. So Conor was readmitted to hospital to see what they could do. He was less than half what his correct body weight should have been.

The surgeons in the hospitals were a little baffled by Conor's condition, as his previous operation should have worked. It was at this stage that they asked a consultant paediatrician to have a look at him and this was when we first met Dr. Margaret Sheridan.

In hindsight I would suspect that the first day she saw him she knew straight away what he had. She asked a lot of questions and did comment that his development was considerably behind where it should be.

A couple of days later I was with my sister Deirdre in his

little room beside his bed when Dr. Sheridan arrived in with a nurse and asked my sister to leave. She told me to sit down because she had something to tell me.

"I SUSPECT THAT CONOR HAS WILLIAMS SYNDROME," is how she said it.

I knew by the look on her face that this was not good but I had no idea what it was at that stage. She proceeded to tell me briefly about the syndrome. She believed that Conor had the facial features that were common to most Williams people and that, compounded with the other symptoms like the feeding difficulties, severe constipation, constant crying, delayed development both mentally and physically—need I say more— led her to believe that this is what he had. She told me about the FISH test, which would definitely confirm Williams Syndrome.

I can honestly tell you that being told the news was the biggest shock of my life. That day the bottom really did fall out of my world I was so heartbroken. I felt this indescribable sense of sadness and utter despair. I was suddenly so terrified of the future and the not knowing what lay ahead of us. I felt embarrassed that our baby was not perfect and that somehow I was a failure. Why had this happened to us? Why us? Why now? I had no idea what to say to anybody. I just wanted to hide away and not have to face anyone, not have to answer anyone's questions as to what was really wrong with Conor.

The one thing that she had said that had stuck in my mind was that there would be some degree of mental disability. My child was going to be Mentally Handicapped.

I can't begin to tell you how much that hurt me. Every time I looked at Conor I felt such rejection towards him. It's all I could think of. I was so disappointed that all our hopes and dreams for Conor had, in the space of a couple of minutes, been changed utterly. How were we going to tell people this? How were they going to react? Would they love him any less? Would they treat him differently now?

I felt so bloody angry with everybody and everything. All I wanted to do was to cry and be left alone to get my own head around it. I was utterly devastated. I was numb. My stomach was sick. I just did not want to believe that this was true.

This is the kind of thing that you see on TV or you read in the papers—but does not happen in real life—not in mine anyway, or so I thought up to this point.

But the truth of the matter is that it does and, like it or not, you somehow have to find a way to accept it in your heartbroken heart and remember that he is still your little baby—the same baby that was yours before you knew what he had. He still has to be loved and cared for and looked after like any other little boy.

It was such an awful time and one I will never forget as long as I live. It is probably best described as the day that had changed my life forever and the lives of all our family.

For weeks and months after I was told I was still really struggling to come to terms with Conor's condition and, if the truth be told, even up to one year later I was still having some really bad days. I just could not seem to see beyond the next day. Every day was torture. I cried every single day, very often on my own so nobody could see how I was really feeling. If I met someone and began to tell them about Conor's condition or someone stopped me and asked me about Conor I just could not help myself—I would start crying—and, as much as I would try not to, the tears would always come.

Every day those words "Williams Syndrome." It was all I thought of night and day. It was driving me crazy. I began to think that I would never be able to accept that my beautiful little son was going to be different from all the rest and would almost certainly always be dependant on myself and Martin.

I found myself thinking of 20—30 year's time. What would he be like then? Would he have friends of his own or would he be some kind of a social out-cast? What level of independence would he ever reach? What would his capabilities be? Would he ever have a real job? Would he ever drive a car?

All these questions, nothing but questions and very few answers. Wait and see is what they said. It depends on what level of the scale he is at. He may be in the mild, moderate, or severe range. Nothing but time will tell us how bad his Williams Syndrome will be.

In truth I was wishing his life away and not at all living in the moment and realising that he was still a 6-month-old very sick little boy who desperately needed us to be there for him. Believe it or not, it is true what they say—that time is a great healer.

On looking back at that terrible time in our lives I feel so sorry for our little daughter Aoife who, at this stage, was 2 ½ yrs old. She knew that Conor was very ill and we told her what Conor had. I remember she asked me when will he get better and when will his Williams Syndrome go away? I felt that I was almost overcome by this unending sense of sadness that would just not go away and, even to this very day, I still have days when I still feel this sense of sadness but not as often now thank God. It does ease as time goes on. I feel I completely fell apart for her and, for the first time in my life, I had to face up to this huge challenge, the biggest so far that has come my way and I just felt that maybe I was not up to it.

This is how I reacted to the news that Conor had Williams Syndrome and I don't know if this is a normal reaction or completely over the top but I didn't know any other way. I really don't think that there is a right or a wrong way to react to news like this. I do think that trashing out all those feelings and emotions is very important. Also, grieving over what I saw as such a huge loss, almost like a death in a way, did help ease the pain and, in time, the emotional distress does get less.

In a way you just have to get on with your life and move forward with what you've got. I always remember my brother Enda telling me in his straight "to the point" way—"You can't keep crying about it, Fiona. Just get on with it." Sometimes you need somebody to almost give you a kick in the behind to knock some sense into you. I had to snap out of it and stop feeling sorry for myself because that's probably who I was feeling most sorry for all along.

We spent nearly three months with Conor that summer, from May until July, in Our Lady's Hospital for Sick Children in Crumlin. We hardly ever left his side. It was very hard trying to juggle Aoife, work, home and hospital all at the one time. Our families were great and were so supportive from the day we told them and still are to this very day.

I decided to give up work completely—a decision that was made quite easily in the end—to look after Conor full time. I have never regretted this. It is probably the best decision that I have ever made and our whole family has benefited from it since that day.

I just wanted to get Conor home so much, to try and get some normality back in our lives. We needed routine and order instead of total chaos and turmoil.

Conor's feeding difficulties did not improve and, in fact deteriorated. He completely refused to take either bottle or solid food in any shape or form. He was wasting away in front of our eyes and we both felt so helpless. The doctors inserted a tube up his nose going down into his stomach {N.G. TUBE} to try and feed him but most of this was being vomited up any way. They then tried to feed him intravenously to build him up again.

My worst memories of this stage were listening to his screams and howls when the doctors were trying to get a vein for the drip. He used to go absolutely hysterical and very often they would have to abandon their efforts and try again later.

Sometimes they would go at him 3 times a day looking for blood or a vein.

He was very traumatised by the whole thing and I really hope that this will not have any long-term effects on him.

Conor absolutely hated the N.G. Tube in his nose and spent most to the day trying his best to get it out. Sometimes he would pull it out 3 times a day, which meant it had to be reinserted again and again, which traumatised him even more. It was such a vicious circle. These were such terrible dark days for Conor and had to be the worst time of his short life so far.

Time moved on and finally we were allowed to take Conor home. He still had the N.G. Tube in his nose. We were trained in the hospital to reinsert the tube into his nose if he pulled it out, and pull it out he did! Conor was just not able to tolerate this tube and, in my opinion, it was the start of a lot of problems e.g. head rocking, tactile defensiveness, etc. There were so many evenings I remember crying and sobbing to myself that I had to inflict this kind of pain on Conor while trying to reinsert the tube into his nose.

As it became clear to us that Conor's feeding was not going to improve it was obvious that we had to start looking at other solutions for his own quality of life and for our sanity. The feeling of utter desperation I felt I just cannot describe. I was so desperate for help and so unsure of what kind of a future lay ahead for Conor I can honestly say that I was beginning to wish that I was no longer around.

Conor was admitted to hospital again with a severe bout of bronchitis and he was finding it very difficult to breathe. He spent 9 days on nebulizers, which had very little effect on him at all. It took a lot out of him and it took him a long time to get rid of this virus.

We plodded on until August 2001 with the NG Tube in his nose and finally, on 18th Aug 2001, he had a gasterostomy fitted. It was to be the best decision we had made for Conor so far. Finally things started to get better for us.

Conor no longer had this tube in his nose and we no longer had the worry and fear of him pulling it out. We finally could see his beautiful gorgeous face that no longer was obstructed by bandages from ear to ear in an attempt to keep in his nose tube.

A gasterostomy is a button placed on a child's stomach making an entry through the stomach wall. You attach a tube to this button and feed the child through the tube, going directly into the stomach and so avoiding the mouth altogether.

It just meant that I was no longer spending most of the day trying desperately to get Conor to feed through the mouth and shoving a spoon in his face every other minute.

All his bottle feeds were going through the tube and, for the first time in his life, he was actually getting all his daily nutritional requirements without me having to go near his face at all. It took so much pressure off and it was at this point that I would say that Conor started to show the first signs of progress. Once his nutrition was corrected everything seemed to follow after that.

Conor himself began to relax and was not so upset and crying all the time. The constant pain he was in seemed to have gone away and he began to smile at us for the first time since he was born. Up to this point Conor had never smiled at all; this was one of the things that used to really bug me—he would never smile, he only cried.

He now has the most endearing and beautiful smile I have ever seen. He began to really settle down for us. His sleeping pattern was becoming more normal and even his severe constipation was improving immensely. We actually saw him as a normal little baby for the first time since he was born.

The gasterostomy was definitely the turning point for Conor. I feel that he has never looked back since. I would highly advise anyone who is experiencing the same feeding difficulties that we were with Conor to seek advice about a gasterostomy.

He began to get really alert, playing with his toys and moving about the floor. His physiotherapist came every 2 weeks and he was showing some real signs of progress.

There was light at the end of the tunnel after all. We began to see normality and routine return to our lives and as life seemed to be getting a little easier for us I would say that, for the first time since he was diagnosed, I began the first steps of trying in my heart of hearts to accept that Conor had Williams Syndrome.

Time was moving on and it was coming close to Christmas and Conor's first Birthday.

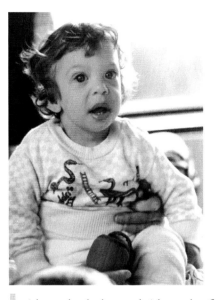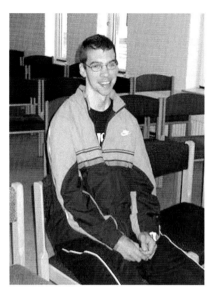

Alan, the baby and Alan, the fine young man.

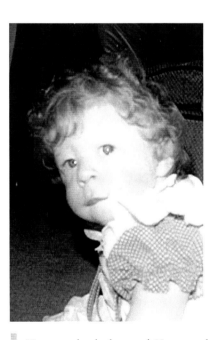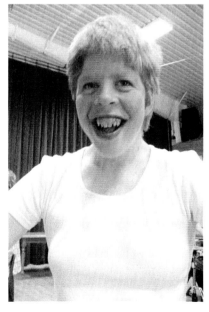

Karen, the baby and Karen, the happy young lady.

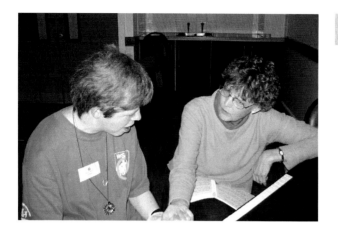

Karen at piano class during the WSAI Music/Activity Camp.

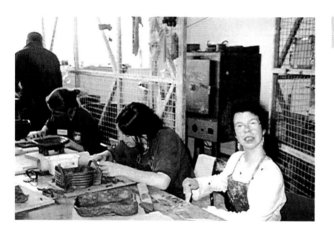

Patricia shows her skills at pottery during the WSAI Music/Activity camp.

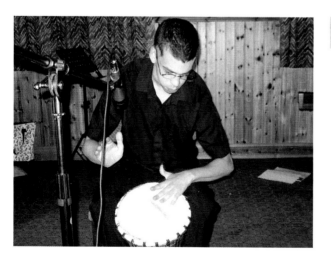

Alan entertains on the African Drum.

Karen concentrating on her favourite pastime.

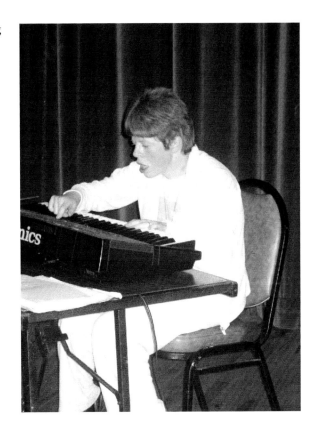

Brian tries his hand (very successfully!) at the drum kit.

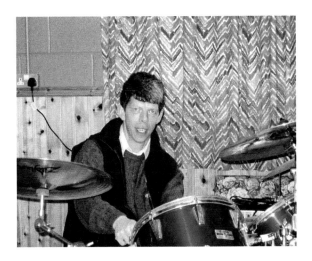

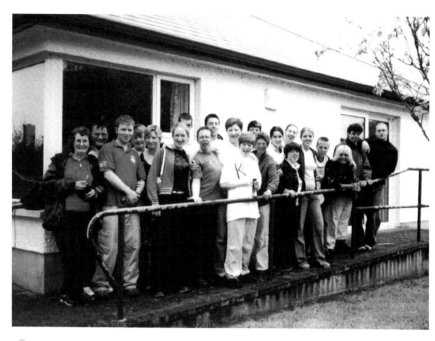

Some of the WSAI group at the WSAI Music/Activity Camp in the Share Holiday Village.

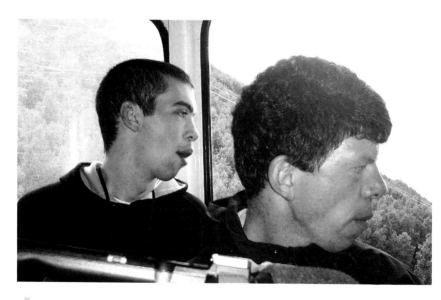

Alan and Brian enjoy the view from a cable car during the FEWS camp in Norway.

On looking back, my husband Martin was cool, calm, solid as a rock, a shoulder to cry on. I sometimes couldn't believe how well he had accepted everything and just wanted to move on with life while I completely fell apart.

However I'm sure that outwardly as much as he showed strength and courage for me inwardly it probably was a different story but he never once let me see that side to him. I'm sure he had his moments on his own where he cried too at his loss and the unknown ahead. He was always so positive. He always said things would be ok; everything will be fine in the end. He never looked at the negative side; always the positive.

Thank God he was there and was as strong as he was and still is. It was really his attitude that eventually made me sit up and think to myself that there was no point in whinging and crying over it. I had to accept it, learn about it, and try my hardest to get on with my life.

On 13/12/2001 Conor celebrated his first birthday. We had a little party for him and I felt so proud of him that day. He had been so ill for the first year of his life and here he was, 1 year on, sitting proudly in his high chair playing with all his new toys and smiling away. He looked so happy and jolly which really is Conor's trademark to this day.

It was becoming clear even at this early stage that Conor had a huge preference for toys that lit up or made any kind of music or any thing that he got a response or a reaction from. They really helped improve his concentration and attention span.

It was coming up to Christmas week 2001 when we got a call from Our Lady's Hospital in Crumlin to take Conor in immediately. As a result of a routine blood test it was discovered that Conor's calcium levels had become dangerously high. He had developed a condition called Hypercalcaemia, which is common in Williams children. It needed to be brought under control as soon as possible.

He was admitted to the hospital again and was put on a special formula called Locasol. This is a low calcium feed to control hypercalcaemia and it eventually brought Conor's elevated blood calcium levels back to an acceptable level. This condition will hopefully resolve itself but lifelong abnormality in Calcium or vitamin D metabolism may exist and will always have to be monitored.

I suspect that this is what was causing Conor's pain and discomfort and made him very irritable. However, once this was corrected Conor became a totally different child to the early days. He is now one of the happiest and most content little boys that I know. He has the most fabulous temperament that you could wish for. He is still on this formula to date, which has worked extremely well for him.

We started to learn a lot more about Williams Syndrome, what it is and the best way to deal with it.

Williams Syndrome is a rare genetic condition estimated to occur in 1/20,000 births, which causes medical and developmental problems. WS is not caused by anything the parents did or did not do either before or during pregnancy. We know that most individuals with WS are missing genetic material on chromosome #7 including the gene that makes the protein called elastin (a protein which provides strength and elasticity to vessel walls). It is likely that the elastin gene deletion accounts for many of the physical features of WS.

Some medical and developmental problems are probably caused by deletions of additional genetic material near the elastin gene on chromosome #7. The extent of these deletions may vary among individuals, so they could have a mild, moderate, or severe syndrome.

In most cases, the individual with WS is the only one to have the condition in his or her entire extended family.

We made contact with the WS Association of Ireland, which was to prove to be very helpful to us indeed. It provided us with lots of information regarding the syndrome and it gave me a chance to talk to other parents of WS children. It also gave me a chance to see for myself WS people at all ages of life, which I found to be very helpful and comforting.

I had so many questions for the Association I just did not know where to start. It took me a long time to contact the association but when I finally got talking to another mother in the same situation as me I have to say it was a huge sense of relief.

The lady I first spoke to was Ann Breen who is the secretary of the association and was also its founder in this country. Ann was so good to speak to. She said so many things that I could immediately relate to. I couldn't help feeling that at last I was not the only one who had gone through this. Ann informed us of the Associations AGM date and location and invited us to come along. She did tell me that there would be some Williams people there and to be prepared.

I have to be honest and say that I was extremely apprehensive as to what I would see and how I would feel at finally seeing and meeting another Williams person.

I didn't know if I was ready for it yet or maybe it was too soon as my emotions and thoughts of the whole Williams Syndrome were still at a very delicate stage.

The day of the AGM came and we had a 2-hour journey to get to it. I was so nervous going down in the car but as usual my husband kept reassuring me that it would not be that bad. To be honest I had this enormous sense of dread as if I was going to see something horrible but I could not have been more mistaken.

We walked into the room where the meeting was and I instantly could pick the Williams people out. Now I could see what they mean by the Williams features. There were four Williams people at the meeting. I just could not help myself. I could not stop looking at them. I watched their every move to see if I could notice anything about them and to see if they were really that different from people their own age. I tried to get to talk to them all—just to see how well they were able to converse with me and conduct themselves. I was so curious and fascinated all at the same time.

I was so pleasantly surprised with all of them. They were all so lovely and instantly struck me as being very happy individuals. Yes, it was obvious that there was some degree of delayed development with all of them but not to the extent that I had imagined and had read about. All four of them were leading fairly full and active lives. Three of them had various jobs and one was still at school. I got talking to their parents and asked many questions about every detail of their lives. All the time I was comparing them to Conor.

The parents all adored their children and it was obvious that these kids/adults were very special individuals to all concerned.

The parents all expressed the same doubts and concerns that I had. Some of them had terrible stories to tell and some had fabulous stories. The one thing that I remember especially from that meeting is one parent saying to me that the earliest days, and getting over the shock of it all, are the worst, but you must accept it and get on with your lives and things will get easier from there. She was so right!

I realise that the longer you go on torturing yourself and living in denial of the whole thing, you are setting yourself up for such a big fall. Because when they don't talk and don't walk at the normal ages and then you have people asking you "Why?" "What's wrong?" it can only lead to huge disappointment and further stress.

We went home from that meeting feeling very positive and more hopeful for Conor's future. I felt that you get out of these kids what you put into them. The more love and attention you give them the more they shine. I have attended many meetings since and find them very fulfilling and rewarding.

Conor's feeding is still a major worry for us, however at the same time it is improving. He is at the stage now where all the solid food he eats through his mouth has to be liquidised to a smooth texture. He has not yet mastered chewing lumpy food. All his bottles go through his gasterostomy on his stomach. We can only hope that as time goes on his overall feeding will improve to the extent that he will no longer need his gasterostomy. He now eats his breakfast, dinner, and tea through his mouth and has a very broad range of foods that he likes. I would definitely say that the only way I got him to eat was to give him very strong tasting foods e.g. Lasagne, Bolognese, curries, beans, fish, spicy chicken, etc.

As the months have passed us by and as I write this story Conor's age is 2 years 4 months and his development is best described as slow but steady. From the moment we got his nutrition sorted he began to develop in every area.

Physically Conor started to crawl at 16 months and standing at 20 months. He was furniture walking and walking holding onto one hand at 25 months, which is all considerably slower than would be considered normal. He is not yet fully walking on his own but is not far off it. Conor's physiotherapist calls once a month at this stage and she is pleased with his progress. She describes his movements as free flowing and confident.

I'm so looking forward to the day he takes his first step on his own. I think I'll be so happy I'll throw a party or somehow mark the occasion. This will surely be a huge milestone for Conor.

Mentally Conor would also be considerably behind his own age level. It is strange because I think he's doing really well until I see another child his age, or even considerably younger than him, seeming so much more advanced.

Even though Conor is 2yrs 4 months I would put him at a mental age of 1 year 4 months. However, we do know things will be slower with Conor and we just have to try to find his level and go with it.

I find occupational therapy very useful indeed. Since our O.T got involved we have seen a huge improvement in Conor's abilities. His attention span has improved so much that he can really concentrate and persist with things until he gets them working or doing what he wants them to do. He needs lots of repetition to show him how things are done but he seems to be picking things up a lot quicker now. He just seems so much more tuned in. Again I will say that as his nutrition is so good it has really stood to his development, but he still has a lot of catching up to do.

At the moment we are very happy with his mental development.

We have had Speech and language involvement with Conor. His speech is very limited at the moment. His only words are dada—NaNa—and some vowel like sounds. However his comprehension is very good. He understands certain things that you are asking him and will respond to these commands accordingly.

We are aware that all Conor's milestones are somewhat delayed but we are expecting this anyway. However we seem to be going in the right direction at the moment with him.

At present, Conor's health is excellent. His hypercalcaemia is completely under control and has been on all of his tests for the last year. He never suffers from constipation anymore.

His sleeping pattern is excellent, sleeping all through the night from approx. 9.30pm to 9.00am in the morning and very rarely waking up.

His blood count is checked regularly and has also been perfect each time it has been checked for the last year.

Year 2 of Conor's life has been so much better than year 1 for everybody concerned and he is now going into his 3rd year of life. He is much healthier than he has ever been. He has blossomed and grown into the most adorable little boy.

He is so undemanding and is no trouble at all to mind. Apart from all his medical issues he is the most content and happy little boy that I know. He hardly ever cries anymore and when he does we know that something is wrong. He has the most fantastic smile that can just light up your day and he is so affectionate.

I cannot put in writing how Conor has affected our lives in such a positive way. When we first found out what Conor had we were devastated and thought it was the end of the world, I really thought that our lives were going to be somehow destroyed by this horrible syndrome. It really is not as bad as it seems in the beginning. He is probably the best thing that has ever happened to me. I adore him so much, as we all do. It's his personality—he is like a magnate and everyone is drawn to him and we just cannot help ourselves.

Even his sister Aoife just adores him and plays with him so well. She has so much time for him and knows he is very special to us all.

I cannot wait to see his happy smiling face in the cot every morning and the way he cuddles into my shoulder is so comforting. The welcome home he has for his Daddy, the excitement he expresses when he sees his Nana and the way he goes into hysterics laughing with Aoife. There is a smile on his face when he sees his cousin Jack and how he watches them play! The fascination he shows when he sees Barney on TV, his total attention and enjoyment when his favourite tape plays. The way he loves to roll around on the bed with Aoife. The way he is so cautious about taking his first step. I could go on forever because we just love him so much.

I feel so guilty now for the way I carried on in the beginning and the rejection I was feeling towards him. How could I have ever thought those thoughts? Now I feel I would die for him this second. I just want to take away any pain he ever suffers from. I would do anything for him.

In the beginning it all seemed so terrible and the future at that point seemed so bleak but we got through it as a family. If anything, it has made us so much stronger and more united. I will be honest though. I still have bad days when I just feel sad about the whole Williams Syndrome thing. I don't feel sorry for myself anymore. I feel sad for Conor. I feel that his future is going to be very uncertain and hard for him.

However, I also feel that with so many people looking out for him, loving him, teaching him, and working with him it can't be all that bad. There is so much more out there now for people with disabilities, whether it is mental or physical. You have to really push for the resources to help your child but they are there. If I were to give anybody, who maybe just found out that their child has Williams Syndrome, a bit of advice, I would say, "Do your grieving the way you see fit." There are no rulebooks telling you the right or wrong way to react. There is no right or wrong way. Everybody reacts differently.

It is such a hard time to experience that only people who have gone through it can understand how it affects your life.

You must try in your heart of hearts to accept it as soon as you can because denial can only lead to so much disappointment and heartbreak.

Once again I'll keep repeating it "its not as bad as you think it's going to be," at least it wasn't in our case anyway. In fact, the last year has been the most rewarding and fulfilling in my life. These children are so loving and bring unquantifiable joy and happiness to a family. You will live and breathe for this child as you would for all your children.

In my case I was very lucky. My husband was, and still is, a huge support to me. He refused to be negative and he made sure he kept my mind focused on the here and now and not to be worrying about 20 years time. I would say that something like this could actually make or break a couple. Well, it certainly was the making of us.

I would never change Conor for what he is. He is our son, our Williams Syndrome son and we are so proud of him for every little milestone he has achieved to date.

I look to the future now and I know that there will be more worrying and hard times ahead. However, I also know that Conor will continue to enchant us all and we have many happy times to look forward to as well. We will do our utter best for him. We will always be here for him.

Our aim or goals for the future would be to make him as independent as possible with a good quality of life but, most of all, my wish for him is for health and happiness.

Billy's Story

When my husband and I were expecting our first child, I was very sick. However, she was born a perfect little baby and we never looked back. When we were expecting our second child, I was very sick again for the nine months but thought it was a repeat of the previous pregnancy and everything would be alright.

When Billy was born he was very small - 5 pounds 6 ounces - and suffered colic. He didn't feed very well and I knew there was something wrong. For the next nine months it was hard with him not taking food, trying to get his wind up and no sleep. We brought him to doctors but they couldn't tell us if anything was wrong. We brought him to specialists but they couldn't tell us much either, only that Billy seemed to have a mild handicap. At the age of four, Billy went to a special needs school and was there until the age of seven. He was better than most in the school so he was moved to a class for slow-learners in another school. Even though he got on fine, he never learned to read or write. He was always acting

97

older than his age. As he got older, he always wanted to work and he had a thing about diggers!

We had two more sons after Billy and we treated the three of them more or less the same. As they got older and our two younger sons started going out, we couldn't let Billy go. It was hard on him and on us. He couldn't understand why his younger brothers could go to town and he couldn't. I think that was one of the hardest times in our life, realising that he couldn't have a life like the rest of them had. We got through it and, when Billy got a bit older, one of us would drop him to and collect him from the village where we live. People here are very good to him and look out for him. He could go to parties and into pubs with music. He would play his jews harp which he loves. He even played with Simon Casey!

Billy had a normal life. He learned to cycle a bike. He learned to swim and he's a very good swimmer. We brought him and his sister and brothers to the zoo every year and to the seaside in Galway, if the weather was nice. He played with his brothers and sister but didn't play with other kids. He would call into the neighbours' houses for tea and a chat. They were always good to him that way.

When he left school, he went to the tech for a year, and then on to day care. They got him little jobs so he wouldn't get bored. When he was in his early twenties a doctor sent him to a Dublin hospital and that's when we found out he had Williams Syndrome. We had no idea what that was and I remember thinking at the time that maybe it had something to do with his name - Billy (William). One day I saw Ann Breen on the television talking about Williams Syndrome so I rang the number and the Williams Syndrome Association was so helpful and asked us to meet up with them. I must say we really enjoyed ourselves. We knew we weren't on our own. We had so much in common with everyone there. We got some very helpful information. Billy loves meeting up and making new friends.

When Billy was twenty-six, he started to complain about discomfort in his stomach. I brought him to his GP, who referred him to a Surgeon in Tullamore General Hospital. Following a series of tests, Billy was diagnosed with diverticulitis and he was prescribed medication and put on a special diet. By the time he was 27 years old, he had been in and out of hospital many times. Then one Sunday night he got very ill. I brought him to hospital and he had an emergency operation. He ended up having to have three-quarters of his bowel removed and requiring a stoma bag.

His life changed, as the bag had to be emptied five or six times day and night. Wherever we went we also had to ensure that we brought spare bags and a change of clothes. I felt that I could not let Billy go anywhere, just in case anything happened and his ileostomy bag leaked, as my husband or I would have to be there to tend to him. We had a hard time with this but, with the help of family and the day-care, we got through it.

I later read some information on Ileostomy reversals and found that many don't work as the person may subsequently have to go to the toilet many times during the day and night. Billy's surgeon advised us to have the reversal done (i.e. Ileo-Anal Pouch Operation) and he felt that Billy would be able, with exercises, to control his bowel movements during the day, although incontinence might be a problem during the night. To get things clear in my head as to what type of operation was proposed for Billy, I contacted the "ia Ileostomy & Internal Pouch Association" here in Ireland and obtained literature from them which was very helpful.

While visiting Billy in hospital, I looked at my son and wondered if I was making the right decision. The next day he was going for an operation and I had no idea if he was going to be better or worse after it. It was a hard decision to make, but if we didn't give Billy the chance we were never going to know. So Billy went down for the four-hour operation. He got through it and, thank God, he was home ten days later. Billy's surgeon, Dr. Rayis, did an excellent job.

Billy was driving a mini digger the day after he came home from hospital and that weekend he was singing at his cousin's wedding. He continues to enjoy a full life and has no trouble with incontinence day or night. I am so happy we made the right decision and we would like to let other people, who are in this situation, know that the operation does work.

Billy has his down days but, thank God, he has a lot of good ones too. Billy gets on well with people and everyone has great time for him. He loves to have a laugh and to hang around with his friends. Billy likes being at home and around the village. He's not one for travelling. We brought him to England to see where the diggers were made. We were in the factory for three hours and he had a great time. But he didn't like the plane! After all he had been through, my husband and I got him his own mini digger which he loves. He is well able to manage it. He would let his sister go on it but gave his brothers a hard time because they were younger than him!

Billy likes to have his breakfast at exactly ten o'clock in the morning. If the bus to work is outside around that time they have to wait until he's finished. He also has to eat at eight and ten at night. He has his own mobile phone and rings home to let us know where he is and where he is going. He's very independent. He got a laptop for Christmas and is well able to use it. With the help of his digger books he looks up all about diggers. He looks up music too, especially Steve Earl who he's going to see in November with the day care unit.

We have four grandchildren and Billy thinks the world of them. They have great time for him too and they tell him that he is their favourite uncle. He visits a lot of people in the village and he has a lot of digger friends and friends in the council and hospital. To them and all his family and friends, we would like to say thank you for being there for him and for looking out for him. It means a lot to him and to us. He couldn't have the life he has without all of you.

When we were young Billy would boss our two younger brothers around because they were younger than him. He wouldn't say anything to me because I was older. When our younger brothers got taller than Billy (and me), he couldn't understand why they were taller than him since he was older. Billy won't eat white meat like chicken and turkey because he says it turns his hair white. Kenneth, his brother, asked him if he eats red meat will that make his hair red and he told him not to be so stupid! Another time we were going to Athlone and Mammy said to him 'isn't that a grand little digger?' Billy looked over and said that it "wouldn't dig worms for a fisherman" it was that small! He was down in our aunt's house one day and was standing beside the telly. He said a bad word and our aunt said 'Billy, holy God is looking at you'. Billy looked over at the picture and said 'no he's not, he's watching telly!' There was an ad on the telly for coal one time and the ad said 'I have a real coal fire' and Billy said 'They're stupid, they can't have a cold fire, it's hot!'

We were brought to the bog when we were younger to rear the turf. Billy would do anything but the turf. He'd go off and talk to anyone that was there. He'd come back either when we were finished or going home. If he didn't like doing something he wouldn't do it.

Mammy and Daddy had, and still have, great parties for him. They had one for his 35th birthday this year. It was packed and we all had a great night. People really make an effort for him which is great. It makes his life for him.

I know growing up we fought like everyone else but the four of us are very close. I know my younger brothers and I wouldn't let anyone say anything bad about Billy. We had great times growing up, laughing and playing and I wouldn't change that for anything. Billy would say something that would have us in the knots laughing. We were at a party one time and this fellow that slags Billy off came in. Billy gives it back though. They let on not to get on but they do. He came in and one of our friends said to Billy 'I hear that fellow's building a house' and without even thinking about it Billy says 'he couldn't build a bird's nest!' All we could do was laugh. Mammy's sister got a gold cap on her tooth and Billy kept staring at her. He eventually said to her 'you have a thumb-tack stuck in your teeth!' All she could do was laugh. Billy also loves wrestling and Kenneth is bringing him to a wrestling match for Christmas this year. He's really looking forward to that. His favourite colour is red and because of that, he's a Man U fan. He shouts for Cork except when Offaly is playing.

Billy likes his work and he loves life. Hopefully, it's a good life.

PART 3: BILLY'S WORK EXPERIENCES AND DAY SERVICES

Billy is a bright young man who has a keen interest in the general building trade. He enjoys being treated as one of the lads and the feeling of belonging to a working-man's team. At present, Billy has work experience every Wednesday in Tullamore hospital. He is assisting some of the maintenance men doing light repairs within the health board and some light work within the stores. Billy also has work experience in Rabbitt's hardware store in Clara two mornings a week: Thursday and Friday. His duties there are general tidying and stocking shelves. While in our day services, Billy attends computer classes on a Tuesday afternoon. On a Thursday and Friday Billy enjoys socializing with peers and staff and going out in the local community.

Billy has completed the following:

- On 29th November 2008 Billy successfully completed his Safe Pass Course through S.W.E.E.T.S. in Kilbeggan. This covers Billy to be on any building site.

- Billy has also successfully completed six months work experience with Offaly County Council in the Ferbane area. His duties there were to assist the maintenance men with light repairs to the roads or repairs to council properties within the area.

- Billy was successfully employed by Tullamore Hardware two mornings a week as a general operative doing light duties in the stock room and in the store i.e. tidying and stocking up the shelves. On 9th May, 2009, Billy was made redundant due to down-sizing of the company.

Billy is now available for work experience on Tuesdays and is availing of the opportunity of joining our own maintenance team within the SCJMS Muiriosa Foundation. Billy would benefit and enjoy being one of the lads and doing a bit of light work throughout the Tullamore/Clara area.

Cian's Story

CIAN'S WAS AN IDEAL BIRTH REALLY. I couldn't have asked for better. I arrived in hospital at about 9pm on 15th June 1994 not thinking for a minute that I was in labour. I had had an achy pain all that day and I was 15 days overdue so the hospital suggested I come in for an examination. I wasn't in pain exactly, just uncomfortable and this had not happened in my previous two pregnancies. I was examined and told that my labour was well under way - big surprise to me! At about 10pm they broke my waters and Cian was born at 11.40pm, a perfectly healthy baby boy weighing in at a normal 7lbs 8 oz. We were ecstatic! After having 2 girls it seemed incredible to me that I now had a boy. I lay back basking in happiness and looking forward to the joys of mothering a wonderful little baby boy. Both my other children, girls, had been relatively easy and I had so enjoyed those early years when they were tiny. Motherhood had always been a joy to me and even the dirty nappies, night feeds, colic didn't thwart me. I loved it all. I was now looking forward to a repeat of all that.

Cian cried loudly straight away and didn't stop in all the time in hospital. He hardly slept and would not feed. I breastfed my two daughters and wanted to do this again but he refused to latch on. In the end, out of frustration and tiredness, I gave up and tried bottles. This was not successful either but at least I could hand him to a nurse while I tried to get some sleep! We managed between us to get some liquids into him by feeding constantly and we were discharged on day four despite the fact that he had lost a considerable amount of weight even by then. I knew that there was something wrong at that stage but I was told that he was just a slow feeder and that it would improve. He continued to cry constantly.

At home we tried every kind of bottle we could find and every brand of formula. I remember squeezing the bottle into his mouth, force-feeding him little and often, with the result that feeding times ran into each other night and day. It was unbelievably difficult and tiring but we persevered and he put on weight at a very slow rate. I continuously spoke to the public health nurse and the GP about my concerns for Cian but was fobbed off that he would improve and just to be patient. We were told that it was just colic and it would pass with time. I was very patient but I was very concerned. I am from a big family of 11 children and had already had two children of my own. I had never seen a child like this. I knew that something was amiss but it seemed that no one believed me. The public health nurse tried to convince me that I was just a worrier and that he was a normal "boy". One day, she insisted that I put him down on the floor, in the middle of the living room and to ignore his crying and make myself a cup of tea. I flatly refused to do this, of course. She suggested that I was unable to cope, maybe depressed, and even that I was spoiling him. Luckily, I knew that none of this was true and I soldiered on for a while, hoping that eventually someone would believe me that this was not normal. Feeding was such hard work and I felt that if I stopped trying so hard and let him lose more weight, then they would have to listen to me and investigate why. But, obviously I couldn't do that to my baby. I since heard of other WS babies who were tube fed and think that perhaps that would have been much better for all of us.

Cian cried constantly. He was very rigid and hard to hold. It was like he didn't want to be held and it gave him no comfort. I wondered was he autistic.

When, at three months old, Cian had made no improvement and hadn't yet smiled, he was referred to Temple Street Hospital for investigation. Apart from the lack of interest in food, he suffered from constipation and had an umbilical hernia which lasted well into his first year. All his "milestones" came late or not at all. He started to smile at 4 months, at about 9 months he was able to sit alone, he crawled at 1 ½ years and stood for the first time at 2 years.

The sleepless nights became almost intolerable. We would take it in turns to sleep in a separate room with him so that at least we would have some sleep every second night. Some nights one of us would keep him in the buggy and walk him up and down for hours on end so that the other would get some sleep and so that Aoife, just a toddler then, would get some sleep too. Our GP suggested Vallegran to make him sleepy which sort of worked but we found that he was generally very bad tempered when waking up after having it. Our GP also suggested sleeping tablets, for ourselves, as we were getting no sleep but neither of us wanted to go that route.

Cian had every test known to man and we were consistently told that he had mild development delay but no-one could explain why. His hearing was tested at regular intervals as if this was the main culprit. In fact, his hearing is fine. We were told at about age 2 years that he had a heart murmur caused by pulmonary branch stenosis.

Despite the fact that tests showed classic symptoms of Williams Syndrome e.g. hernia, hypercalcaemia, stenosis, very poor appetite, repeatedly bringing up feeds, and development delay, he was not definitively diagnosed until he was 2 ½ years of age. This came as a complete shock to us. Up to then we always imagined that whatever was wrong could be "fixed". I will always remember the exact moment we were told.

Around that time, I was coming to the end of my tether. I felt let down by the hospital as they were telling me nothing. I had just found out by accident that he had a heart murmur despite the fact that this had been noted in his chart a full year before (I took a sneaky look at his file when the nurse wasn't looking). One day I rang the hospital in complete frustration and demanded to see the paediatrician. I told his secretary on the phone that I wanted all the information on my child's condition and that I wanted it immediately.

I remember the paediatrician sitting us down and straight away telling us that Cian had Williams Syndrome. That meant nothing to us. We had never heard of it. When we asked what that meant all he was able to tell us was that he would have a very low IQ and that he would never go to mainstream school. I think we were so shocked that we didn't really take it in and, in a way, it was a relief. I think we also subconsciously believed that, now that we knew, that we could do something about it. Once he was diagnosed and put on a calcium free diet he improved immensely, both physically and in terms of well-being. He started to slowly put on weight and was much happier. He began to become affectionate and started vocalising more.

We went to great efforts to find out more about the condition but there was very little information available about it, apart from the bare minimal facts about the physical characteristics. We decided that we would do our best for him and that we would ensure that he was given whatever help he needed. He was going to be fine.

At age 3 years he started to form some words e.g. 'Ma', 'Da', 'all gone'.

He was referred to St Francis Clinic in September 1997 for assessment and speech therapy. From then on we considered that he progressed very well. He started to play with toys (cars were always his favourite), began making appropriate sounds (e.g. car engines), was energetic and playful and generally was very happy and affectionate. He was still very small and immature looking for his age.

The clinical psychologist at St Francis Clinic informed us that at age 36 months Cian's development age was 18 months but, she admitted that he was very unco-operative and disinterested at the test and that she could not state this definitively. She further advised that his weakest area was in speech and language. He was referred to St. Vincent's in the Navan Road.

Our main concerns about this time were his feeding, speech and sleeping. Reflux and vomiting continued well into his teens.

It was around this time that we first made contact with the Williams Syndrome Association. I suppose up to that time we were sort of in denial and hoping that he would be "cured" though we knew and understood what WS was.

One evening I got a phone call from my sister who told me to quickly turn on the TV to BBC. There was a programme on, Mind Traveller, and it was focussing on Williams Syndrome. It was a real eye opener for me. The programme was great and focussed on the positives but, of course, I just picked up on the negatives. It was the first clear picture I got about the condition and what it really meant to have WS. It really upset me. For the first time I realised that this was for life. Cian was not going to be cured. I cried for the rest of that evening and then the next day I rang the Williams Syndrome Association and spoke to Ann Breen. She was brilliant. She spoke of her own experience and told me all about her lovely daughter Karen. She didn't give me too much information, just the amount that I needed at that time and she suggested that I attend a weekend away that she had organised for the following March. I will always be grateful to her for her understanding and sensitivity and just for being there. Over the years the Williams Syndrome Association has been a tremendous help and support to us.

Cian was first assessed by a psychologist in January 1998 when he was three years old. A second assessment was carried out in April 1999 when we were considering primary school placement options. This encouraged us to place him in mainstream school and we enrolled him in St Mochta's in Clonsilla. This was our local school and our daughter Aoife was already attending there. We wanted them to be in the same school so that they could have each other close by. We were assured by the school that he would have access to a resource teacher and would continue to have speech therapy through St. Vincent's. In actual fact, it emerged that we would have a battle on our hands to achieve any of these resources for Cian.

Cian's sleeping pattern has always been very erratic and remains so. When small (up to about 5 years old), if left to sleep on his own he would cry constantly, getting so upset that he would vomit. This was very upsetting for all of us so I would lie down with him until he slept. A habit was then formed where he would sleep in our bed, which actually worked very well. He continued to sleep with us until about age 6 or 7. To this day, he is still a very bad sleeper but rises early in the morning. This can sometimes leave him tired and despondent during the day but despite this, he still sleeps badly at night. Today, at age 15, he is sent to bed at 10.00 pm but usually remains awake for some hours. Up until age 14 he still liked to sleep with me, his Mum.

His diet is still very limited, consisting mainly of chicken nuggets, pizza, chips, peanut butter sandwiches and yoghurt and he drinks only apple or orange juice or blackcurrant squash. He eats no fresh meat, cheese, eggs or vegetables apart from a few carrots.

In general, we were happy with Cian's progress in St. Mochta's Primary School and have not regretted the decision to send him there. He was always happy in school and made good friends. He is very sociable and he got on well with his teachers and his peers. His behaviour has never been a problem and he understands the rules and all commands put to him. There are, however, a lot of disappointments in the progress he has made academically. Although we were assured that he would have access to a resource teacher, this did not happen until he was almost 8 years old. We also were given the impression that he was entitled to a classroom assistant. Eventually, after a battle with the Department of Education, he got one in first class but only for 3 ½ hours per week. In fact, it wasn't until 4th Class that he was given a full time SNA.

Speech therapy was also very intermittent. In fact, during his whole time in primary school he only had about 4 sessions, each lasting six weeks for one hour per week.

We feel strongly that, had Cian been given proper resources in primary school together with speech therapy, he would have made excellent progress. As things stand, we are disappointed with his progress, especially in the area of reading. His writing is a little better and he has a reasonable understanding of numbers and is doing simple sums. The main thing, though, was that he was very happy in school and this kept us going when things got tough.

It also helped greatly when we were faced with the decision of where to go from there, when he was approaching the end to his primary education. We had to make a decision about secondary schools. We were greatly assisted in our decision by the resource team in St Mochta's. We all agreed that socially Cian would be well able to cope with mainstream secondary school and, at that stage, his happiness was our priority. We had to consider, however, that he would find the curriculum difficult and that, as he got older, the gap between him and his peers would widen and this might present difficulties. After much trepidation, a lot of discussion and soul searching, we decided to send him to the local mainstream secondary school. They were very accommodating and, in the lead up to his starting there, they met with the resource team in his primary school and were very accommodating to his needs. They also arranged for several advance meetings with us and St Mochta's and some of these meetings were attended by the SENO and the psychologist at St Vincents. I cannot praise them enough for the way they prepared for Cian's introduction to secondary school.

Cian is now in second year and he loves it. Yes, the gap between him and his peers has broadened but they are very good to him and have always made him feel welcome in their activities. He is still very slow academically but he is making some progress. It remains to be seen how he will get on as his peers become more focussed on their exams but we are adamant that his happiness is paramount. If we see any deterioration in that then we will do whatever is necessary to ensure that he continues to blossom even if it means changing his school.

What we want for Cian is that he can read and write adequately, that he has good knowledge and comprehension of maths to allow him operate effectively and independently in time, but most of all, that he can reach his potential both socially and in the workplace when he reaches adulthood.

Cian is quite physically active. He loves swimming and is a member of "Phoenix Flyers", a Special Olympics swimming club. He also attends a Special Olympics sports club where he plays soccer and basket ball. He has won medals at national level in basketball and swimming.

Music is also his passion and he plays drums. He listens to a wide variety of music from Westlife to Slipknot. The highlight of Cian's year is the WSAI music camp which he attends every year.

Like any boy his age he plays too much play station and watches too much TV. He is very competent on the computer and often puts me to shame in how quickly he can navigate the internet.

He is a wonderful boy and a joy to be around. His smile and demeanour light up a room and he gets on well with everyone he meets. He is chatty and friendly, perhaps too much so at times.

I have to admit that at times, especially when he was much younger, I wished that Cian was "normal" and didn't have Williams Syndrome but now I realise that that is part of what he is and we love him so much just for being him.

Donal's Story

Donal was born on 10TH November 1987. He was our first child. We were delighted as, after two miscarriages and a threatened miscarriage with him at 8 weeks, it was a relief to finally have our son.

We had been living in London since 1985 and, as he was the first grandson, everyone in Ireland was happy for us, especially our parents. I had given up work when I was 2 months pregnant after being advised to take bed rest. Donal was born in St Thomas' Hospital and was 10 days overdue. He was 7 lbs. 3 oz and was a normal delivery. He had a head of black hair - Mohican style - and a small button nose.

He looked OK. I breast-fed him for a couple of days but it was very difficult as he just wouldn't feed and cried quite a bit. The nurses suggested I bottle feed him instead. He was still a difficult feeder and had to be fed little and often, every two hours.

He was checked over by a paediatrician and everything seemed fine except his hips. They called an orthopaedic surgeon, Mr Mike Smith, to check him out. He told us that Donal had dislocated hips, seemingly common in Irish babies. He was put into splints. He also told us that his hips would probably rectify themselves in three months. I had seen other babies in Ireland with this problem before who wore double nappies and were ok eventually. I took him home after five days.

It was very awkward. I couldn't dress him properly because his legs were stretched out as if he was doing the splits. We had to dress him in clothing for an 18 month old. He cried a lot and never seemed settled.

We took him to Ireland at 15 days old for my sister's wedding. I was her bridesmaid. He was very unsettled and we put it down to the stress of travelling. He still continued to cry a piercing cry and never seemed to settle after the little amount of food he would take. I thought it was because of his hips and the fact that he was uncomfortable.

He looked thin and pale and started projectile vomiting after every feed. He had his six week check-up. They seemed happy enough with him even though he wasn't gaining weight. They told me I was over anxious about him as a first time mother and not having my family nearby when I told them that he cried constantly and vomited after every feed. I was feeding him Milumil milk at this stage.

I took him back to St Thomas' Hospital to see Mr Smith, the orthopaedic surgeon, at 12 weeks. He removed the splints but didn't seem too happy with his hips, particularly his right one. It still clicked in and out. He said that they would keep him under review as baby bones don't show up on x-ray until 12 months.

He had all his vaccinations and check-ups at the health clinic every few weeks and still wasn't gaining weight. He cried morning, noon and most of the night. I was at my wits end and getting nowhere with the doctors at the clinic. They dreaded to see me coming.

One evening while changing him I noticed a lump under his tummy button. I rang my mum in Ireland and she told me that it was probably a hernia. I took him to the clinic and they confirmed that it was an umbilical hernia. They said that it didn't need any investigation or treatment at that time but advised me to keep his nappy high and tight over it.

His feeding and crying got worse. He still wasn't gaining weight. After numerous trips to my GP and health clinic, and constantly being told to relax with him, I decided that enough was enough. One Friday afternoon I decided to take him back to St Thomas' A&E Department. I waited for two hours before they eventually let me see the paediatrician. He examined Donal from top to toe and told me he had a heart murmur and was very under-weight. He gave me Gaviscon liquid and told me to give it to him before every feed and to bring him back the following Monday if things did not improve over the weekend.

Nothing changed. I sat him up most of the time, day and night. I was more exhausted than he was. Back I went on Monday and he was admitted straight away. He was under the care of a paediatric consultant named Dr Colin Stern. He was checked from head to toe and they were amazed that they had missed his heart murmur at birth and again at his six week check-up. They tried feeding him for 24 hours as I had done at home but it didn't make any difference. They started tube feeding through his nose as his stomach was almost closed from lack of food and he was dehydrated. This was difficult as he constantly pulled out the tube. They did numerous tests on him and decided that he was just a faddy eater. They put him on Prosporal and also a thickener through his feed so that he couldn't vomit. This helped as, once he had his bottle, it would set in his stomach and there was no way he could get sick. It was horrible stuff but it worked.

He was seven months old before we started spoon feeding and that was a battle. He hated everything off a spoon except mini yogurts. We struggled on, with very little sleep. He would sleep for ½ hour and then wake up for hours. At night he only needed 4 to 5 hours sleep.

When he was 15 months old he had an operation for a

squint in his eye and was checked regularly by an optometrist. At 18 months, the orthopaedic surgeon decided to break his right hip and to put a plate in because the splints used at 3 months of age hadn't worked. This was hard as he was in a plaster of Paris from his chest to his toes for six weeks with only a tiny opening for his nappy. He had not walked before this but he was just about ready to start. It was also difficult because he had to be flat and had to be turned every hour. He had to be dressed on top only in clothes for a 3 to 4 year old. He couldn't go in the buggy or car seat. After six weeks the plaster was removed. They had broken the ball of his hip joint and turned it into the hip socket. The plate stayed in place for 12 months.

He walked at 23 months. He was still a bad eater and wouldn't chew anything. Even to this day, he doesn't like lumpy or hard food that needs to be chewed. He is not a great eater of meat. He was being reviewed in St Thomas' Hospital at this time.

At 2 ½ years, Donal was referred by Dr Stern to Guy's Hospital for an ECG and a check-up by another cardiac paediatrician. After the ECG was done, I wheeled him in to meet the consultant. He looked at Donal in the buggy as I walked in and asked me how I was coping with a Williams Syndrome child. I looked at him, bewildered, and said that he must have the wrong notes as this was Donal Carroll with a heart murmur and hip problems. He said that Donal had the facial features of a child with Williams Syndrome. He described the condition - bad feeder, projectile vomiting and fear of loud noises. He was describing Donal to the last detail. He then showed me a photograph of a child with Williams. It could have been Donal's twin.

He told me to get in touch with the Williams Syndrome Association in UK and gave me the phone number and address. I was totally shocked. I was then 3 months pregnant with my son Brian. I told him this but he told me that he was not aware of any family with two Williams Syndrome children. He said that I could have a scan every month to see if there was any problem with the heart and that, if there was, I could have a termination. They had no other way of knowing if something might be wrong. I opted for the scans but termination was not an option for me.

The cardiac surgeon at Guy's Hospital was amazed that, after 2 ½ years, we had not been told by Dr Stern or the staff at St Thomas' Hospital about Donal's Williams Syndrome. He organised for Donal to have a cardiac catheterisation done to check out the narrowing of his heart vessels. This was found to be very mild.

It was hard being told that Donal had Williams Syndrome but, on the other hand, it was a relief to have a name for what was wrong with him after all the difficulties.

We contacted the Association in the UK and they were very helpful. I went to the AGM and met with Ann Breen and Marian Ryan from the Irish WS Association who had been invited as guests.

When I got Donal's next appointment for the paediatric clinic at St Thomas' Hospital, I went along to meet Dr Stern and his team to question him about Donal's condition. He was shocked that we had been told about Williams Syndrome by another hospital. When I asked him about the diagnosis he couldn't answer except to say that he didn't think that we could have coped had he told us when Donal was a baby. He told us that Donal did not have hypercalcaemia and that Williams Syndrome was difficult to diagnose. I refused to accept this and left the hospital disgusted at the way we had been treated.

After scans every month, Brian, our second son, arrived with no problems, thank God. Donal was now 3 years old. He attended a mainstream nursery and seemed happy enough until one morning he got out and was missing for two hours. He was eventually found by the police on the top floor of a tower block. He loved climbing stairs but he couldn't climb back down. From then on, and even to this day, he is very cautious on stairs or escalators.

He was assessed by a psychologist and started in a special school. He had speech therapy and occupational therapy. We didn't find the school very helpful as the teacher was near retirement age and all the children were taught as a group regardless of ability.

We discovered by accident that a family with a Williams Syndrome son lived 100 yards from us in the next road. Their son, Terry, became great friends with Donal and to this day both our families are very close. Terry is 5 years older that Donal and his mum, Karen, became one of my best friends. We still compare notes and offer each other advice.

When Donal was 5 ½ years old we decided to return to live in Ireland. I got referral letters from St Thomas' Hospital to Dr Desmond Duff in Crumlin Children's Hospital in Dublin. Donal was seen there and they were happy with his progress. We had to have him re-assessed there as they wouldn't accept the reports from London. This took time so he was 6 years old before he could start school.

He started in Scoil Chormac Special School in Cashel. He settled in very well. His Principal, Mrs Shannon, was very good and available at any time. He stayed in that school until he was 18 years old, having moved on to the senior school when he was 12. He got on well with all the staff and with fellow pupils. He was involved in all their drama shows and also sang solo with the choir for communions and confirmations.

When Donal was 12 years old he developed a limp. After a lot of investigations and x-rays, he was referred to Dr Fogarty's orthopaedic clinic in Crumlin hospital. They discovered that he has no socket for his right hip. This would explain why the splints and surgery as a baby didn't work.

He was being assessed yearly with a view to constructing an artificial socket and hip replacement eventually in Tallaght Hospital.

He was also seen by Dr Fergal Quinn in Crumlin when he was 13 years old to have his kidneys checked out. He has always had to go to the toilet once he had anything to drink.

They discovered that he has a very small bladder and were prepared to do reconstructive surgery to correct this with a permanent catheter. We decided against this as it was major surgery. It would have been very traumatic for him as he has a phobia of needles, hospitals and alarms. We have learned to live with it.

Donal finished in Scoil Chormac when he was 18 ½ years old and started in the Moorhaven Centre in Tipperary Town. He travelled there for 2 ½ years doing life skills, computers (Fetac), woodwork, drama and horticulture. He is still there in the Sheltered Section. He has done a lot of the same courses and has also done work experience in a gym, restaurant and a pub.

Donal has been involved in Special Olympics since 2000. He has competed in the Munster and Ireland Games in athletics, golf skills and bocce. He was on the Munster bocce team in the 2010 Ireland Games in Limerick.

He also attends the Williams Syndrome Music Camp in Fermanagh every year and loves getting involved in the shows and making friends with the many young people who help out there.

In early 2009 Donal developed a skin condition called Morphea on his neck. It is a very rare condition which causes skin pigmentation. There is no treatment for it but it has to be protected from the sun.

Donal was diagnosed with Type 1 diabetes during Christmas 2009. We found out that he had very high blood pressure and he was put on a 24 hour monitor. As a result he was prescribed blood pressure tablets. The hospital was also concerned about his kidneys failing.

The diagnosis was a major upset for him and for all the family. It is random and effects people between the ages of 4 and 30 years. It was extremely traumatic as he was in Limerick Regional Hospital for 4 days on drips and injections. He now has to have insulin injections twice a day and has to have his blood sugar levels tested 3 to 4 times a day. His diet is very restricted also and this is very difficult as he doesn't understand the consequences of eating the wrong foods. His whole world has been turned upside down so abruptly, especially with his phobia of needles, but, as always we will have to get on with what life throws at us. Donal is a very sociable young man and hopefully he will accept his diabetes in time.

I have made many good friends in the Williams Syndrome Association and also in Special Olympics because of Donal. He has brought us much joy with his achievements and, please God, this will continue.

I want to dedicate this story to my parents who were a fantastic help to me always with Donal - from summer holidays, when we lived in the UK, to keeping Donal during the summer so he could attend a Special summer camp in Nenagh. Mum is no longer with us but Dad is still there with advice or help at the end of the phone.

Thanks, Dad, for everything.

Elva's Story

AM I NORMAL? This is a question that my sister Elva asks from time to time. How do you answer that? Well, normal means 'standard' or 'usual' and Elva, just like anybody else, is not a 'standard' person. She has an unusual name, a unique personality and a beautiful spirit. Elva also happens to have Williams Syndrome but she does not like to be defined by it or any other tag that people ascribe to her. So no, she is not normal – none of us are!

Elva is 1 ½ years older than me so we have always been close. It has not always been easy to have a sister with WS, just as I'm sure it was not always easy for her to have a little sister that acts as an older sister. Elva used to constantly bite and pinch me when I was very young. It's only in latter years that I recognised she was taking her frustrations out on me. We shared some great times in our room together, making up games, playing with dolls and singing songs. Elva had lots of quirky little ways as a child – a fear of grass, vacuum cleaners and thunder. She still makes little balls of shredded tissue. But she was my big sister and I turned to her when I needed her. When I was settling into Montessori school, she came and spent time with me there. I was so proud showing off my big sister. We protected each other. I was so protective of her that I got into a few fights defending her when other kids would make fun of her speech. Those nasty comments would make me so angry. It also used to frustrate me when others would tell me off for squabbling with Elva, as if I should treat her differently. I don't feel as guilty now as I used to for squabbling with her - she's my sister so, of course, we fight. All sisters do – it's normal.

Elva has been through a lot in her life. She had major heart surgery at the age of 6 and I vividly remember having to be gentle with her and mind her because of this. She was in and out of hospital when she was young. I used to enjoy tagging along to all the speech therapy sessions and check-ups. I sometimes resented all the special treatment she got though. Elva could do no wrong as a child and I often got the blame for things she did! Dad was recently astounded when he found out that Elva had lied to him about something. I have known she was a proficient liar for years!

Elva wasn't diagnosed until she was 9 years old. Dad sat me down on the stairs and told me she had WS. I didn't know what it was and didn't really care because she was the same as she always was. The only thing I wanted to know was whether that was the reason she had no tears when she cried. I still don't know the answer. Having a syndrome does not answer every question.

Now that I'm older, I understand Elva better and I understand myself better as well. As a child and teenager, it can often be hard to reconcile the feelings you have and the feelings you should have. I felt guilty if I didn't do things with her. I felt all eyes were on me to see how I interacted with Elva and her other school friends. I felt compelled to volunteer at a social club in Elva's school, even though I was a painfully shy teenager. Although I did enjoy it, I always felt like I didn't do enough and that I should be more of a crusader. Now I realise that I don't need to be a crusader. She's my sister, not a project.

Elva and I have entered a new phase in our lives. She's now in her thirties and I've moved away and got married. We still see each other several times a week but now we're not under each other's feet. I'm incredibly proud of all she has achieved. She works part time in a restaurant in the airport and goes bowling every Friday. She has a great sense of humour and gives us all a great laugh. She is quite independent, although I worry about her when she heads off on her own on the bus or the train. She has WS quirkiness – her life is ruled by time, she religiously writes in her diary every night, she's obsessive about Meatloaf and she gives a lot of hugs. She is such a huge influence in my life and has undoubtedly shaped me as a person.

I feel incredibly lucky to have Elva as my sister. She doesn't need a label. She is what she is.

James' Story

In January 2002, when my husband and I realised I was pregnant with our first child, we were very excited. I had an easy pregnancy and birth. 10 days late, our son James arrived on 5th October at 13:44. He was 7lbs 1 oz and 20 inches long. Our world was complete. We could not wait to take him home and start our lives together as a family.

When James was born the doctors noticed that he had a heart murmur. Although this is common, because there are heart problems in my family they wanted a cardiologist to see him. The appointment came for November, when he would be 5 weeks old, to attend Crumlin hospital to see Dr. Duff. However, James was sick when he was 2 and a half weeks old and attended Crumlin hospital at that stage with vomiting and diahorrea. He came home after 4 days and was back in with a hernia when he was 4 weeks old. They sent him home saying they would operate on him when he was 6 weeks old. By then he had double bilateral hernias. We attended Dr. Duff when he was 5 weeks old. He was vomiting again and the doctor asked us could he get some blood tests done to see what was happening with him. At this stage we did not realise how serious this was but we were afraid to think that something was wrong and what that could be.

James was christened on Sunday, 10th November. We had a great day and he was well, although he had not slept day or night since he was 2 weeks old.

The day came for James' operation on the hernias. He was admitted fasting for surgery. The operation went well but James had a high temperature afterwards so they kept him another day. The nurse told me to strip him down to his nappy, to turn off the radiator, open the window (it was November 21, and quite cold outside) and to leave him in the cot to get the temperature down.

A few minutes later, Dr. Green came in and told us that one of the blood tests that Dr. Duff had asked to be done (it was the F.I.S.H test) showed that James had Williams Syndrome. He explained a little bit about it to us, most of which went over our heads, gave us a leaflet and asked us had we any questions. I asked would James be able to have children. He said genetics have come a long way in the last 5 years and who knows what will happen by the time James grows up. I looked at my child wondering what did all this mean.

The nurse came back in to take James' temperature and we told her. She said she knew nothing about this but said "don't forget he is the same child you brought in here on Tuesday". I had been fighting my feeling to pick him up because I was told to leave him in the cot to get his temperature down, but I picked him up when the nurse left the room. My husband James and I huddled in a corner of the cubicle - a room that all of a sudden seemed so big - not sure of what lay ahead but very sure about the love we felt for James.

We spent the next couple of weeks explaining the little bit of information we knew about Williams Syndrome to other concerned people and trying to find out more about it and how to help James. We contacted the Williams Syndrome Association of Ireland. Ann Breen posted me some information and told me to contact her again whenever I needed to. We arranged to meet at the gathering of the Association in Fermanagh at a musical week the following August.

But, ultimately, we were dealing with knowing our baby had a disability and we did not know how mild or severe this was going to be for him. Sometimes the reaction of other people helped lift our spirits for a while but every night was hard because James did not sleep. A crying baby and sleep deprivation are very hard to cope with when all is well. When you throw in a syndrome, it makes you feel you are alone in the middle of the night and this carried on for 14 months. James did not sleep during the day either. He cried most of the first year and a half of his life. I did not go back to work. I stayed at home to help James as much as I could (I probably would not have been able to work with exhaustion anyway!). You lose touch with the outside world. The only way you keep contact is through your family as they try to keep you going through this. You also lose contact with friends. The only friends you keep are the ones that try to comfort you and have the patience to listen and call you constantly.

We met with the Williams Syndrome Association of Ireland in August. It was enlightening. We learned that life for James was not so bleak. For the first time we could see a realistic future for James. We met one adult with WS who could drive a car. He could also write music. Another WS person could live fairly independently with a little help from her Mam and Dad. This was particularly helpful to us as parents to be able to see what James could aspire to.

We had to try to find out what we were entitled to and then had to "fight" for some of these entitlements. The public health nurse we had in our area at that time was very good to me. She told me about the allowances I was entitled to and referred James to St. Catherine's School for special needs children. James started to attend their clinics in the local health centre from the age of 3 months. Although always in and out of hospital with appointments and admitted for minor illnesses, James was reaching his milestones and mostly passing his development tests until his 12 and18 month development test. He still was not talking much or walking at all. He was not even creeping! However, there were more important things to worry about!

When James was 10 months old, we had an appointment in Crumlin hospital with the cardiologists. James had pulmonary stenosis and aortic stenosis. We were told James' aortic stenosis was very narrow and they wanted to do a test to see how narrow it actually was. James was admitted to hospital on 14 December 2003. The test showed his heart was under immense pressure and that he should not be left too long to have the operation to have the aorta, as it exited the heart, widened. They feared his heart could give out at any stage.

By February of 2004 we had heard nothing about a date for James to have his operation so we contacted the hospital. They told us they were only dealing with emergency cases at that time. As James did not have that chance to be an emergency case - as he would literally just drop dead - we fought to get a date for him to be admitted. His operation took place on 3 March 2004. The operation went well but, when he was in the I.C.U., they could not stabilise him. For 3 hours they worked to try to stabilise him. There was a clot behind the heart causing a problem. They had to clean out around his heart. We were devastated and could not think past this! The nurse came out to us with a key to a private room. I could not deal with this! I could not walk into that room thinking what she was going to say. I turned to my husband and told him "No, there is only one reason you get brought in there!" The nurse said she only wanted me to be careful and that I should sit down. I was 7 months pregnant with our second child and it could be a while before we know how James was. I went in reluctantly. When we were brought into the I.C.U. to see him I had to fight my instincts to pick him up and give him a hug, I kept telling him we were there and that we loved him. The only word James could say was Dada and he kept repeating it and shaking his head. The nurse asked us not to talk to him as she was trying to keep him sedated. Thank God, James recovered well and came out of I.C.U. the next week and home the following week.

After a few weeks at home James started to creep and talk. It was great to see him recovering from such a major operation and getting on so well. This was one of the high points and was very encouraging to us as his parents.

When James' sister Donna arrived on 25 May 2004 he was very gentle and loving to her. He loved to help to feed her bottles and wind her. As they grew up together they bonded very well. As Donna started to reach her milestones I realised how James was different. Donna started to walk when she was 11 months old. James did not like this and, if she stopped near him, he would grab her by the hips and pull her down. James realised she was doing something he could not and this helped to motivate him to do things himself. They get on very well together now, although Donna is the only person James will take his frustration out on. He will go over to her and, at first, he used to try wrestling her to the ground but now he just puts his hand up to her face to annoy her.

James was attending St. Catherine's early learning services once a week where he and I went to the school and took part in a group session for 3½ hours. It was decided to assess James to get a base line for how his development was getting on. When James was assessed in November 2002 he was presenting with a 12 to 14 month delay in all areas. When you are faced with an assessment on your child and it shows he is a 2 year old child with a 1 to 1 1/2 year old mentality, it is very hard to read. You find yourself reading it over and over again and getting very down about it all - as if it is your fault for not being able to help him more!

James started in St. Catherine's Preschool in September 2005. He settled in well and loved the bus journey to and from school. I found it very hard because it was the first time I was not involved with his learning directly. I found myself thinking "he is only going on 3 and has started school". He left home at 8am and did not get back until almost 4pm, I missed him so much. I hated to see him going in the morning but I knew I had to let him go for his sake.

James was only attending the school for about 2 weeks when he got very sick. The doctor put him on clear fluids but a few days later he was getting worse. The doctor sent him to hospital. The doctor there tested him for coeliac disease and appendix failure. After 10 days his hands and feet began to swell. This was due to the albium in the blood breaking down due to lack of food and nutrients. After that, he started to slowly eat and get better. The hospital sent him home the day before his 3rd birthday with strict instructions that we did not bring him out or allow many visitors to see him. James was following the 9th percentile on the growth chart which made him look short and underweight for his age. After his operation he was nothing but skin and bone! It was so hard to look at him in the bath with his sister who was growing at a rapid rate for her age. This was also the first time James had been admitted into hospital since Donna was born. It was very hard having a child in hospital so sick and another child at home - you missing her so much and knowing she was missing you too.

James got stronger and stronger from then on. He was still attending the outpatients department of Crumlin hospital regularly (at least once a month) but he was progressing steadily.

James started toilet training at Easter 2006. He was getting on very well. I had been dreading the idea of it but he took to it very well. He had a slight setback when he got the Chicken pox that June but he trained himself at night after a while. The following March we decided to take him out of the training pants. He loved the freedom of this. However, James started to have "accidents" during the day that June and, by the time the summer was over, he was also bed wetting. Sometimes he would wet the bed 3 times during the night. He had an ultrasound scan done on his kidneys and bladder which showed that one of his kidneys was slightly smaller than the other one. The left kidney also had a double drainage coming from it to the bladder. James still has "accidents" in the day as well as at night. There does not seem to be any pattern to it and it does interrupt the night time in the house. He now gets back into his bed and eventually goes back to sleep or else he keeps coming into our room until he gets into our bed! In order to get some sleep during the night, this is sometimes the only option!

James was assessed again by the psychologist in St. Catherine's in April of 2008 and it was agreed that he would be able to cope in mainstream school if he had the back-up services from the H.S.E. We enrolled James into Balintemple National School in Ballycoog which is approximately 10 kms from our house. There were only 14 students in the whole school, divided into 2 classes. They welcomed him very well in school and encouraged him, taking him into the community.

He completed his first year in school and the only areas that let him down were the handwriting and the physical exercise. He participated and interacted well with the rest of the school. James' teacher was very good with him and his Special Needs Assistant had a great rapport with him. He also received 5 hours of remedial teaching which he loved.

The assessment that was done in St. Catherine's was sent, with our permission, to the H.S.E through the disability act where, unfortunately, he did not get accepted so well! The only therapy he was offered was physiotherapy once every 3 months. I had another fight on my hands, one I was determined to win. I could not let this happen to James as he was giving all he had. I was going to put up a fight for him. I phoned the H.S.E. a few times a month. I posted letters and got everyone I could think of to post letters to them regarding James. They still gave him nothing more. The assessment under the Disability Act is reviewed every year and, when it came to that time, I phoned the Assessment officer. She was aghast that James was given so little. She asked a multi disciplinary team that was initially set up for the under 5 year old children, to take him on as he does not "fit into any group or category". He was receiving no help! They met with us and James and (thank god) they took him on.

James is now receiving a proper physiotherapy service and will be seen by the Occupational therapist and a Speech & Language therapist in due time. The sociologist phones me every week to get an update on James and gives me advice on how to help him. This help for James should give the best possible chance for him to succeed in mainstream school.

James was getting on very well mentally as well as physically until last June. He was looking forward to his summer holidays from school. On Wednesday 24 June, James as usual walked into our bedroom at 4:30 in the morning. He slept in our bed until my husband got up at 6 am. James asked to go with him but I said no. A few minutes later he told me he wanted to go to the toilet. This struck me as unusual because he normally just got up and went. When I told him to go ahead, he turned to me with fear on his face and said to me "I can't, Mammy". I took him up, not sure of what was going on, and stood him beside the bed. He had to hold the bed to stay standing. He was holding his left arm and leg awkwardly. I brought him to the toilet thinking he had "pins and needles" in his left side. When I took him back out, he could not stand or move his left arm or leg. I phoned the caredoc as it was only 6:30 or so. The nurse told me to bring him straight away to hospital and to bring a mobile phone with me. She said that I should ring for an ambulance if he got short of breath.

When we arrived at the hospital we were seen almost straight away. They x-rayed his arm and leg. When they read that all these were ok, they sent him for another x-ray on his hip to be sure. Looking back, we realise that broken bones would have been the best case scenario for James! After lunch the cardiologists saw James. They did an echocardiogram which showed everything was ok with his heart. The suspicion was that a clot came from the heart and James was temporally paralysed when it reached his brain. As the day went on James gradually got the movement back in his leg. The neurology specialist admitted James to hospital. The next day James had a bit more movement in his arm and gradually by midday he had full movement back in his arm and leg. We were so relieved we almost could not believe it. On Friday the hospital had an opening for James to have an M.R.I. scan. Thankfully, this scan showed normal activity in the brain. This ruled out a clot still there, bleeding or a tumour in the brain. Relieved that more serious things were ruled out, we were still concerned as to what did happen and could it occur again and, if so, when. None of these questions have been answered yet! There were blood tests taken from James that evening while he was under an anaesthetic. All have returned a normal result. James was sent home from hospital that Friday night on 1/3 of an aspirin tablet a day and has been attending the G.P and the hospital regularly since. We have just been to an appointment to the neurology department and they are to consult the haematology department to see if James can be taken off the aspirin tablet. As James has not had another incident in almost 6 months, it is unlikely to happen again, although it was very unusual that it happened in the first place.

For my husband and me, our children have been the centre of our lives. From the day James was born he has brought something special into our lives. There have been times when we have felt alone and thought that nobody knows what we are feeling or going through. However, we know that it is a precious gift to have a child like James, especially when he can lift your day with just a smile or comment. It is then you know the meaning of life. Many people asked me when I was expecting Donna if I was not afraid of having another child with something wrong? My answer to that was "no, I was only afraid that she would not sleep". James will no doubt have more problems in the future. All we can do is hope that we are able to deal with them and that we all will be ok.

Jarlath's Story

*"Sunday's child is bony and blithe and
good and gay"*

On Sunday, 27 February 1983, Jarlath was born with a
cacophony of angels announcing his arrival, or, they may
as well have been, considering the incredible joy his birth
brought. An early morning labour for Mam, who went
into hospital at eight and produced a baby boy at ten, was
unremarkable. For her, this birth took the edge off the grief
and sadness of her Dad's death the day before. For four
little girls, aged from twelve to three, the news that they
had a baby brother was the most exciting thing that had
happened. We danced and cheered at the news. We hugged
and kissed one another and couldn't wait to mother this
new baby. We didn't realise just how much this new baby
would enrich our lives and change it forever. My stakes in
the new baby were higher than that of the others despite
the fact that I was the second eldest. The reason for this
was my elder sister Dearbhla had been 'second mother' to
our youngest sister Maeve, a role I resented. I swore with
the announcement of Mam's pregnancy that I would be
second mother to the new baby.

With granda's funeral, it was Wednesday when I got to

school, high as a kite, to announce the arrival of a long-awaited brother. Mam was due home the following day and the wait was almost too much for a ten-year old kid. We were bitterly disappointed to learn that the baby, who was only five pounds at birth, was being kept in hospital for an extra few days. Mam decided to stay there too, needing the rest.

When Sunday finally came, we all bundled into the car to collect Mam and the beloved new edition to the family. We oowed and aahed the whole way home, commenting on his little fingers, his little nose, his little ears ... so small and so incredibly perfect. I made a comment that day that plagued the next twenty five years with guilt. I said to a relation who visited that he looked like E.T. and was told that in no way did my beautiful baby brother resemble that awful ugly alien. It was only when I hit my late twenties and learned much more about Williams Syndrome that I could explain those remarks that had no malicious intent. What I was referring to was in fact the WS features ... the retroussé nose and the long philtrum, the slightly wrinkly area around the eyes and the full cheeks were evident to me when this baby was seven days old. Naturally, with the reception my remarks got, I never referred to it again!

Mam breast-fed Jarlath but, beyond that, there was an army of little girls waiting hand and foot on the baby. He was cuddled and carried, he was sung to and talked to, he was idolised! At age ten my life was consumed by Jarlath but I began to notice things weren't as they should be after about nine months. I was asked by my teacher, who had a baby girl around the same age as Jarlath, if Jarlath was walking. Walking?? My God, this baby was a long way from walking. I said no. He asked if he was standing? Alarm bells! Jarlath was only just sitting. It made me realise that Jarlath was obviously very behind his peers at that young age. I was bothered about it but didn't express this worry.

Of course, when he wasn't meeting his developmental milestones, it was picked up and he was admitted to hospital for tests. Nothing was revealed. Nurses who knew the family told the paediatrician that all the Tynans were small and light-weight. One joked that our grandfather had to have stones in his pocket on a windy day! There was no apparent reason for Jarlath's slow rate of development and it was put down to the fact that four little girls were doing too much for him. He only had to look in the direction of a toy and it was given to him. He only had to open his mouth, not even utter a sound and his needs were pre-empted. His trip to hospital upset me greatly. When he came home he smelled different and I was angry at the world for deeming him to be less than perfect. To us, he was the most wonderful baby. He was incredibly loveable, good natured, placid and settled. He rarely cried, he fed well and he was so damn cute!

At a year Jarlath was moved into my room. We were inseparable. I'd lie down with him at night until he fell asleep and I'd get up with him in the morning. He was a good sleeper and I loved the chance to really become second mother to him. When we realised it might be us impeding his development, we did all we could to encourage him to walk. Jarlath never crawled despite all the cajoling! He was a bum shuffler and could move with incredible speed this way. But he needed to be able to walk, so one of us would hold him by the dungaree straps and another would bang spoons in front of him. He took his first steps when Eimear and I were minding him but no one believed us because he didn't do it again for a while! Few babies in the history of mankind were encouraged as much as him!

Jarlath's love of music was noted very early on. He would sit mesmerised listening to anyone singing. He particularly loved songs in different languages and loved to imitate the sounds which made him laugh. Nursery rhymes and action songs were performed with him. Any songs we learned at school were sung repeatedly to him. At one point 'The Fields of Athenry' was the song being learned. Jarlath's response to this was unusual. The lip went down, the eyes filled up and, if the song continued, he'd cry and get very upset. With this we began to see the effect music had on him. It could actually dictate his moods. He could also hear rhythms in everyday objects and they would hold his attention. He'd dance to the sound of the washing machine. I started playing the violin when Jarlath was four. He would laugh out loud every time I hit a bum note, which was quite often. He'd giggle when I played scales and arpeggios even marginally out of tune and once told a visitor to the house 'Fionnuala's useless at the fiddle!'

Jarlath was also very slow to talk and again the adoring sisters were blamed. But when he spoke for the first time it was an extended sentence. Once he started he never stopped! His fear of loud noises was also noted. He'd cover his ears tightly with both hands when a loud or unexpected noise sounded. It was also connected to anxiety. He'd get very upset on a cold morning if the car wouldn't start. He'd again put his hands over his ears and cry, sometimes doing this before the keys were even put in the ignition. As time wore on we strongly discouraged this by pre-empting his distress, talking him through what may happen, talking him through what was actually happening and physically holding his hands so he had to concentrate on what we were saying. The behaviour diminished and disappeared with time.

As a little fellow who failed to reach developmental milestones, he availed of the services of Western Care. There was a home tuition scheme which was invaluable. It consisted of a social worker who visited the house once a week, did some activities with Jarlath, showing Mam what to do and leaving a selection of materials and a list of activities to be done before the next visit. It was all the usual infant education materials: threads and beads, pegs and pegboards, jigsaws and shape sorters. He enjoyed them, including the jigsaws, which is an activity not normally enjoyed by many with WS. He also did well with them, although in retrospect he was certainly behind his peers in the number of pieces to his jigsaws. He also availed of speech therapy from Loretta, a highly encouraging speech and language therapist. She saw his potential and always told

Mam he would do great things. He would have done anything for her. She found fun ways to do everything.

One area that needed a lot of work was spatial language. We finally cracked it on a trip to France. As we drove to our apartment, several hundred kilometres from the ferry by motorway, Jarlath was sitting on my knees in an era before car seats for children over two were introduced! Every time we went under a fly-by, I'd say 'under the bridge'. I nearly drove everyone in the car bananas but by the end of the journey even Jarlath was saying 'under the bridge' every time we went under a bridge! Sweet success! The 'doing' of the action seemed to greatly help his understanding of spatial language. We didn't really realise his spatial limitations until much later on because he was always outside on a trike or car and didn't seem to have any difficulties with navigating round the corners of the house. He learned to ride a bike without stabilisers, although this took a lot of time. After he learned this skill he lost interest and that was that with cycling!

Jarlath went to playschool at four where he was wonderfully supported. The highly-effective teachers realised his needs and gave Mam lots of advice on helping his development. He stayed for a second year in that playschool because he made such good progress. But the question of his primary schooling was looming. Naturally I was not involved in any of these discussions but it was a scary time.

A psychologist came to the house to carry out some tests. She told Mam and Dad that Jarlath would never ask a question. She was so full of doom and gloom that it made us realise the extent of Jarlath's needs. Of course, she was way off target. This gave my mother an eternal horror of psychologists. The psychologist also observed Jarlath in the playschool environment. At one stage she took him out to a separate room for testing. On the way she dropped a pile of alphabet cards. Jarlath handed them to her one by one after looking at them and said "Here's your p, and here's your x, and here's your a". This fascinated the psychologist. From her observations she didn't think he had that ability and wasn't even going to test him in such things. This shows the 'peaks and valleys' of the WS learning profile that has baffled psychologists for years but also shows how multi-faceted intelligence is.

The results of the report came back to say that Jarlath would benefit from a special education setting. I'll never forget the day. Mam cried all day and, when she told us the news when we came home from school, I felt my world shatter. It felt like once again the world was judging Jarlath as something not quite normal but they were failing to see the true essence of his being which was so bright. I remember going into the sitting room to find Jarlath sitting on the floor in front of the television (to this day he still sits on the floor watching television!) totally unaware of the turmoil happening. He turned when I went into the room and beamed his wide smile and I dissolved in a pool of tears.

I had a big problem with Jarlath attending a special school. I felt a residual guilt that if we had done more as a family with him, if we gave him more time, if we structured activities more we could have normalised him. Of course, we couldn't have done any more with him. From each of us he was given a different energy and skill base.

With Dearbhla he had his social outlet. Every Saturday afternoon he went into town with his biggest sister and met with her buddies in a coffee shop or pub.

With me he had his educational programme advanced. It's no wonder I went into teaching. I'd take the activities that the social worker or speech and language therapist had assigned and do them with Jarlath. I'd spend hours at task analysis, breaking up simple activities into small steps to teach him how to tie buttons or fold clothes. Eimear was sporty and took him outside or to the garage each evening and played football or basketball with him, developing his gross motor skills and hand-eye co-ordination.

Maeve, the closest in age to him, was probably the most normalising factor in his life. She fought with him and asserted her rights as had been done to her by her older siblings!! Despite all the attention lavished on Jarlath, Maeve included him in all her play activities. In older years she included him in her social activities too, particularly those that were community based like Foróige. In so many ways he was spoilt but no one was prepared to do anything about it because 'poor Jarlath' had special needs. He went through a phase of having aero bars as his treat. Without anyone knowing (because I'd have been told off), I'd give him an aero bar in the sitting room and tell him he had to share it. For the first few times he refused so I'd take the bar, break it in half and tell him if he didn't offer it, it would be shared *for* him. He learned pretty quickly to offer a piece of his treats to anyone present, as he ended up with more of the bar for himself that way! But the tendency to spoil him was always there, still is in fact!

Time moved on and Jarlath did well at school. He went from being barely able to hold a pencil in his hand to being able to write legibly. He sometimes got in trouble for lording it over his classmates verbally by using phrases from films or television. I remember calling to collect him from school one day and the teacher called me aside to tell me that Jarlath had called one of the children in the class 'my little pig droppings!" that day. Of course, straightaway, I knew this was a line from the film 'Annie' but the teacher was less than impressed. I was angry with her that she couldn't deal with it and had to be telling me, a sixteen year old, tales about what he did in class.

He always had prominent parts in his school plays or Christmas nativity masses because of his excellent verbal skills. Swimming was part of the school programme and Dad (who was also a swimming teacher) would join the school for swimming activities and help Jarlath, who hated this cold and wet activity. When both myself and Dearbhla were in Leaving Cert, PE was an option. We used this time to go swimming with Jarlath's school and help out, primarily with Jarlath. We also helped Jarlath with fundraising. A big drive was held each December where it was either selling tickets or selling lines for a skipathon. Every year Jarlath won the first prize for raising the most money, mainly because Maeve went from door to door every evening for weeks and bled the community dry! We have photos of Jarlath holding his win each year, an enormous teddy, up to his shoulders!

Reading came quite easily to Jarlath. He particularly enjoyed poetry, word rhymes and Dr. Seuss books. He loved sounds and plays on words. He genuinely enjoyed language. He was read to by all of us at home and there was always someone to listen to him read or test him on his flashcards. As time went on we found he could read well but found comprehension exercises very difficulty. He couldn't recount a story, or sequence it and the detail was often distracting. He fared better when the story was read to him. He seemed to be able to elicit more information that way without the visual distractions when reading himself. But it was so frustrating when he couldn't tell you what had happened at the beginning of a story, or what the main character had just done.

Jarlath was quite successful with maths. He enjoyed working with numbers, in particular. He could tell the time very quickly and mastered the 24 hour clock without any difficulty. He wasn't pushed on much regarding numerical operations at school so never learned subtraction with borrowing or how to do multiplication or division. When he was in his mid-teens his teacher sent me a letter (I was a teacher myself at this stage) and asked me to see if I could get Jarlath to learn tables. I found that by doing them to a rhythm, just tapping it out on the table as I said the numbers, Jarlath picked it up very quickly. But real life maths, like real life skills, was always the deficit. The only way to learn such skills is by doing them, so we're still at that!

Time moved on for me too and in 1992 I was in Leaving Cert. I had decisions to make. I would have been quite happy to have stayed at home and worked rather than leave Jarlath behind. I cried myself to sleep every night of that year at the thought of leaving him. My choices were really centred around

Jarlath ... primary school teaching, speech and language therapy or medicine. I had two teachers at the time myself who were very good to me and knew about my very close connection to Jarlath. They both, at different times, reminded me to make choices for myself and for the long-term. Mam and Dad felt that with all my interests in music, art, drama, and languages, that primary school teaching would facilitate those energies. Leaving to go to Dublin was a heart-wrench but I made great friends who invited both Jarlath and I to their houses at holiday time! It was most definitely the best choice for me. I was a very happy classroom teacher!

In Jarlath's third year of school he had a teacher who really pushed him academically. He made more progress in those two years than we could have hoped for. She researched his behaviours and came up with infantile hypercalcaemia! She showed a great interest in him, not just as a student but as a person. In conjunction with the principal he was given a job to counteract his hypersociability. He had to greet visitors to the school and show them where to go without engaging in conversation! So, in many ways, the school catered for his William Syndrome behaviours.

But I still wasn't convinced that he was reaching his potential. He had a great ear for languages. Dad taught himself French over a period of about seven years, from when Jarlath was about four. They'd sit in the office for sometimes hours in the evenings, the pair of them, singing French songs. It was a shame that in Jarlath's school no language was on the curriculum, not even Irish. Jarlath really had an ear for the grammatical structure of Irish. It was so developed that even the local school inspector mentioned it to me when he realised I was Jarlath's sister! When Jarlath was about 15, the school in which I was teaching was included in a foreign-language pilot project for primary schools. Because of Jarlath's interest in languages, I managed to include him in our language lessons. Since it was me that was teaching French to my own fifth class, it required minimal discussions with others.

I collected him each Wednesday lunch time. He had about fifteen minutes of play time with the children in my class who were aged 10/11. He had a half hour of a French lesson with me and my fifth class and then another half hour French lesson with me and sixth class. It was a really good experience for me to see firsthand the WS behaviours in the classroom. Jarlath has a tendency to wander so this needed to be curbed in the classroom. His attention was also very poor but he was alert when learning language through songs. When it came to reading and writing activities he was quite far behind and couldn't keep to the pace. He also lost interest quickly when the material got too difficult. What I found more than anything was the benefit for my pupils. For many of them, this was their first encounter with special needs and it was such a positive one. I was so proud of Jarlath, so proud to be his sister. My kids were mad about him, as were the other teachers in the school. For Valentine's day, he got a card from every girl in the class! For Christmas they all clubbed together to get a selection box for him! And to this day when he meets any of those children (now adults!) in town, they always stop to talk to him and call him by name. But what I got out of that experience more than anything else was I could put to bed the guilt that if we had worked harder with Jarlath as a baby he could have made the grade to attend a mainstream school.

When Jarlath was 14, the Oliver Sacks documentary on WS was shown on BBC. A cousin of ours, a psychiatrist, was watching and phoned straight away saying 'this seems to be what Jarlath has'. This was 1997 when that internet age was only dawning in Ireland. I went into Castlebar library with another cousin of mine who was adept at ICT and typed in Williams Syndrome. Lo and behold, pictures downloaded and text appeared and there could be no question but that this was what Jarlath had. It answered all our questions. I had a voracious appetite for any WS information. We were relieved that none of us were 'carriers' of WS as we wondered if there had been more boys in the family would they have had the same needs as Jarlath. Most importantly we found out no one is to blame for a WS occurrence. A microdeletion at the moment of conception meant there were no guilty parties.

I contacted the Williams Syndrome Association and downloaded information from every WS website I could find. Jarlath found this a very difficult time. He associated Williams Syndrome with Down Syndrome and was less than impressed that he was labelled. After a brief connection to the association, Jarlath refused to be involved for a number of years and then when he became curious about his condition himself, we became involved again. He understands that he's missing genetic material and once in the car said to me 'if only I had that vital ingredient'. He mourns the fact that he's not 'normal' as he sees it. Despite repeated conversations that we all have strengths and weaknesses he knows better. He regrets that he never had a 'debs' like the rest of us, or a graduation with the hat. He notices these things. It saddens me to see him wish he could be something else because we wouldn't have him any other way.

Our next-door neighbours are wonderful and have supported Jarlath at every stage. From when he was a little lad he'd go over and wander into their house, often causing us great distress not knowing where he was. He was always welcomed into their house and they treat him as one of their own. Indeed, Ann was one of the few people who would take Jarlath off Mam's hands for a few hours when she was visiting her own parents, or going into town. Brendan used to take Jarlath for a 'man's day's work' each year during the summer holidays. He's teased and cajoled by them as much as he is at home. As their own children have grown up they are like additional siblings. They were always playmates for Jarlath and they were always extremely kind to him. The most touching act was when Carol, the eldest daughter, asked Jarlath to be godfather for her first baby. It meant such an incredible amount not just to Jarlath but to all of us too.

The night of Jarlath's 21st made us realise how deep Jarlath's aura emanates. Where the rest of us had a family dinner for our 21st due to parents who don't like a fuss (!), Jarlath was not happy with this arrangement and began to invite people to a party. Eventually, six weeks before the date Mam and I decided that we needed to do something about this and we organised a real party! Jarlath made out the list of invitees and we invited the hundred and twenty on the list, old and young, an eclectic mix of humankind. It was a magical night and the excitement was so great that we had a surprise party for his 25th and he's already planning a big party for his 30th! And you know he's right. His attitude is we might be dead tomorrow, life if for living and for partying!

Where are we now? There's no doubt about it but Jarlath has come a very long way. He can read. He flicks through the Irish Times every day. He finds out what's on the television, he gets football scores on teletext, he checks webpages for information on cinema times and the likes. He's a total politics-nerd and won't miss any 'Week in Politics'. At election time he's elated and feeds off the transmissions on results of who is elected and on what count. He has a great general knowledge and has a great interest in the wider world. He has strong views on many world issues, which are not always those of the rest of us in the house!!

Jarlath has a number of social outlets. He's involved in Special Olympics bowling, he has two friends with whom he goes to the cinema from time to time and, of course, he has his sisters. He comes into my house frequently at weekends to stay. He goes to Carrick on Shannon every couple of months to stay with Maeve and he goes on the occasional trip to Dublin to stay with Eimear. He's incredibly attached to his four sisters and finds any break from the family very difficult. Even going to the WS Music camp is a challenge for him. He misses what's familiar and becomes very anxious when his routine is broken.

I tried to get him into a local male choir last year and

was incredibly dismayed at the outcome. I'm very involved in music circles around Castlebar and know many of the members in different groups. When I asked a prominent member of the male choir about Jarlath joining he hemmed and hawed. He asked could Jarlath read music. No. Well, then it would really be too difficult for him, he concluded. Interesting, considering that over half the members can't read music. Even Dad was approached to join the group a few years ago and was told that reading music wasn't important! When I refuted this point I was told that membership was closed for that particular year. So there are still obstacles to be overcome and, sometimes it's so disheartening, I feel like I did all those years ago when Jarlath was a baby. I'd love to run away with him to a desert island and protect him from the ignorant people of the world. But, of course, that would be most damaging to him!

On a brighter side, his love of music was noted by the conductor of Mayo Concert Orchestra. George, the conductor, used to ask at each annual concert if someone in the audience would like to conduct the last piece of the programme: the Radetsky March. Jarlath and Mam attended every annual concert but Mam would never allow Jarlath to volunteer! One year he slyly put up his hand, the hand that was on the opposite side to Mam, so she didn't realise until George was heading towards them with the baton! Jarlath was a natural. He stood in front of us and conducted as well as any conductor could. He turned around to get the audience to clap and indicated to the musicians when they were on the last repeat, showing a very clear understanding of the music. I cried and laughed as I played, I was so proud to be conducted by him. At the end, as the audience stood to applaud him, he took off his glasses and bowed three times to the audience, those on his left, centre and right! What an attention-seeker! He was so good that he has been the guest conductor every year since. That's one of the highlights of his year!

Workwise, things aren't so simple. Services at this stage of his life are also very poor. He works with RehabCare every day but the quality of the service is extremely poor. He is not stimulated and he is certainly not developing any skills. It's an ongoing battle. He did a number of other placements over the years with a rollercoaster of results. His concentration and wandering were a problem when he did a computer course but the biggest problem was that the staff wouldn't involve us at any level in the programme, despite our requests. His placement in Castlebar library was one of the greatest successes. I'm not sure what the library got out of it but Jarlath lived for Wednesdays. The staff members were incredibly caring and nurturing. Jarlath came home every day of his work in the library with stories of who he had met and what they said. But with cut backs and the likes, the chances of a repeat placement are slim to nil.

As a family we have discussed Jarlath's future. We are prepared for changes that will have to be made in the event of something happening Dad and Mam. I attend all meetings for parents so I'm up to date with what is happening on Jarlath's job front. I bring him to his dental appointments and for the first time this year I took over his medical check-ups too. My greatest worry is that, if Jarlath has to live with me, his dependence level will cause us both huge stresses as we adjust. If he were more independent there would be less 'settling in' to be done. As it stands there is no way that I could do for Jarlath all that Mam does on a daily basis.

Our immediate concerns are getting Jarlath to shower independently, to prepare simple meals for himself and to be able to dress himself appropriately (with tops tucked in, collars in place and trouser legs not in socks!). It's the little things in life and none of these things are insurmountable. So far Jarlath is a complete bundle of joy. He is almost always in good form. He sings around the house and always has a smart comment at the tip of his tongue. He rings his different sisters at different times of the day. We are immeasurably lucky that there are four of us to continue to help and support Jarlath to develop and grow into the amazing adult that he is.

We thank our lucky stars that we hit the genetic lottery with him: one in 20,000 births and we won it! And the results of that lottery will be with us for this lifetime.

Kelsey's Story

ON THE BIRTH OF MY SECOND CHILD, Kelsey, there were no complications. It was a normal delivery and I was only in the hospital 40 minutes before she was delivered. No pain relief was used, only gas and air. Kelsey weighed 7lb at birth. We were overjoyed. She was so cute and had a mop of curly hair.

At first, we thought she had colic as she cried a lot and our first born had also suffered with colic for a few months. While we were in the hospital she developed the jaundice and she was moved to the ICU for treatment. We stayed in hospital for 5 days and then went home. We visited the nurse twice a week to check the jaundice and her weight, and went back to the hospital for the BCG vaccination.

It was only at her 6 week check-up that the consultant noticed a difference to other babies. He thought she was underweight for the formula intake she was drinking. When he checked her chest he noticed a heart murmur. He also thought she was a bit floppy. He told us he wanted to run some tests starting with an x-ray and an echo. These tests came back and Kelsey had a slight heart murmur. They also monitored her formula intake. The consultant thought she looked a bit different. He said she had a few characteristics that indicated she had a syndrome.

Curly hair
Heart murmur
Sticking out her tongue
Low weight gain
Floppiness when pulled up by the hands.
Her back passage was very close to her front passage

He said that if each of these characteristics were on their own it would be fine but because they were all together it indicated something. He wanted to do a few blood tests and send them off. Kelsey was released and we went home with the deep realisation that something was wrong, but what? That was the question...... That was May and we got a call from him in early August to say the test results were back and Kelsey had a syndrome called Williams Syndrome. That night we read up about Williams Syndrome on the internet. We cried for a while with the realisation that things were not perfect and wondered what problems we were going to come up against. We went in to see the consultant the next day. He gave us a lot of information relating to Williams Syndrome and set up a few appointments for us with a geneticist in Crumlin hospital. He also gave us Ann Breen's (WSAI) number to contact and talk to.

We went to see the geneticist and he was very familiar with Williams Syndrome. The one thing I remember about our visit with him was that, when we were leaving, he said to us to remember if there was ever a syndrome you would wish for your child it would be Williams Syndrome because they are very sociable, loving and happy children. That stayed with me because he was bang on.

Kelsey's first few years were very busy with visits to the hospitals; she had an eye operation when she was 18 months for a squint in her eye. She had every scan going and all came back clear, thank god. After she turned 1, she was referred to the Sisters of Charity early intervention team on the Navan road, where she was assessed by speech therapists and an occupational therapist. In between all these visits we did get to enjoy her learning as she was very bubbly and happy. She had to work hard to walk - her walking was delayed - and we attended physiotherapy weekly to fix this. Her balance wasn't great. There were times when she would fall down. Her spatial awareness wasn't great either and she couldn't judge the height of things e.g. if she was going from the path to the kerb she would get down on her knees; if she was changing from the concrete path to the grass surface she would get down on her knees. Although Kelsey struggled with walking and toileting, her vocabulary was very clear and she had a lot of words, even though she didn't understand the meaning of all of them.

With the early intervention services, we were assigned a community nurse who came to visit once a week to help with Kelsey's early pre-school learning. We worked on the portage scheme where she would leave an activity for Kelsey to work on for the week. Repetition worked well with Kelsey. We would work on her gross motor and fine motor skills. Kelsey found it hard to ride a bike or to hold a crayon. From an early age, we noticed she had a love for music so we would often sing to her to help with activities or bang out commands against the table. Kelsey would hear a song once and remember the tune. She still surprises us with the amount of songs she can sing.

We found it hard to find a suitable play group for her to attend and, when I did find one, we were told we didn't qualify as we didn't live in the parish and we were not disadvantaged. We enrolled her in a local playgroup for the first year and got on to the local TD to ensure she had a place in the more suitable play group for the following year. It worked! We were offered a place the following year. It was the making of her! They supported us in the toilet training and, within a month of attending, Kelsey was fully toilet trained. There were now only eight children in her class and the previous year there had been 20 children.

We also had problems trying to get her into special school. We made an application for a school for children with mild to moderate learning difficulties. Our application was not accepted as only 7 places were available and there were children on the waiting list longer than Kelsey. We applied for mainstream; the school was very enthusiastic about taking Kelsey in. The psychologist recommended that she have a fulltime assistant and learning support. We made our application with the psychology report to the SNO (special needs organiser). We were granted a part time assistant and no resource time. We went to see the local TD again and chased it through him. He brought the issue up with the minister for education. We were granted a full time class assistant but no resource time. When we got in touch with the SNO she told us that if Kelsey had Dyspraxia she would be granted resource time. Although Kelsey had trouble with her motor skills and spatial awareness, she did not have Dyspraxia! When she started school, she was delighted! She was well loved and looked after although she did have a few clashes with the boys in the class. When this happened, she was just taken out of the class and brought on errands. She would not go into the hall for shows or assembly. She didn't like the piano playing in the hall and she would get upset. We re-applied for the special school and lodged the issue once again with the local TD.

We were told in April that she had a place in the special school for the following September.

September arrived again and another school - her fourth, to be precise. The only difference this time was that we knew she would be there until she was 18. She settled into P1 well and loved the teacher. After about three months, we were called in to be told our child had behaviour problems......... Kelsey had a habit of biting her hand and she would clash with the boys. She was the only girl in the class during the first year.

An appointment was to be made to see a behaviour psychologist. We were put on a list for about two years. In the meantime we tried working with the school to try and improve Kelsey's behaviour in class. Kelsey is very sensitive; she can go through every emotion in a five minute period. Kelsey attended an art therapy course in school where she would discuss her feelings. In her second year of school, the teacher moved schools and a new teacher started. This upset Kelsey and it unsettled her as well as her whole class.

The teacher only stayed till end of term. Another September arrived and a class move to P2 and an experienced teacher and assistant. We also got word of an appointment with the psychologist.

Stan and Kelsey and I went to the meeting; Stan and I were interviewed and asked about our family life and Kelsey's behaviour at home. We were sweating after it. We were scheduled in for 6 sessions. Kelsey found it hard to express her feelings and this is what we worked on. The psychologist visited the school and tied in with the staff there. She felt that they needed help in understanding children with Williams Syndrome. Things have since improved with her behaviour in school.

Kelsey loves music and her school have encouraged her with her talent. The music teacher takes her twice a week. At Christmas she sang on her own and did a duet with her friend in her class. Although Kelsey loves music, she suffers with hyperacusis (over sensitive hearing) which is also related to Williams Syndrome. We could be in the car driving and she could be singing in the back listening to radio and all of a sudden she would be screaming hysterically. Certain noises, tunes, instruments and motors can set her off. The Hoover used to be a major problem at home but now she accepts it, as long as the flat part is left on. The kids know when it is going to happen and they alert us by saying "ears". We joke that she can hear the grass grow but it wouldn't surprise me if she actually could!

Kelsey is well known in the community because she is

involved in a lot of after school activities and because she is very sociable. She goes to gymnastics on Tuesdays and Saturday mornings. This has helped her with her balance. On Tuesdays she goes to a Special Olympics swimming club and on Saturdays she goes to the Brigins. During the school holidays she attends a camp in the local gym with children aged between 5 and 12.

I haven't mentioned before that Kelsey has a love for food! She eats most types of food as long as it's not too spicy. At this stage we keep a lock on the fridge because she could over eat and she doesn't realise she is full until she feels sick. We used to have terrible problems when she was younger with her getting sick from over eating. Kelsey loves to go to restaurants and loves cookery programs.

Kelsey has a love for animals and would be able to give information on a wide variety of animals e.g. where they live and what they eat and what their babies are called.

She loves all books on animals and she remembers most people's pets and their names.

Our house is always lively and that is because of Kelsey. She is a character. Life is one big party to her. While out playing with friends, she often invites them all to dinner or lunch and we get a knock on the door and a few hungry heads looking up. If there is a new movie release to the Disney channel we have to have a party. When she goes to bed it often takes her an hour or two to go asleep. When she does, she sleeps all night now. When she was younger we were like zombies walking around! She used to wake 5 times or more a night.

Every morning - rain, hail or snow - she marches into the bedroom with "rise and shine, it's a beautiful day". She never gets up in bad form. Kelsey is so good at music and rhyming that she surprises most people!

The WSAI Story V

JULY 1994. The family membership is growing. There are now 22 WS families on the mailing list. The WSAI held its first weekend outing in October last year. This outing was to Trabolgan Holiday Centre and was very successful. The families that attended gave very positive feedback so we hope to run this as an annual event going forward. The next outing is being planned for March or April 1995 and we hope to continue at that time of year thereafter.

We are also starting to organise informational seminars to be run in conjunction with the AGM of the WSAI each year. This year's speaker will be Dr Neil Martin from the UK who has years of experience of dealing with WS children.

At about this time, I begin to notice articles in the WS Association magazine about the musical abilities of Williams Syndrome people. I had already noticed the musical interest in my own daughter, Karen, and had also heard other parents attach the same interest to their own children. The parents in the USA had started an annual weeklong music camp to encourage and develop this musical interest. I began to wonder if we could do something similar in Ireland. The main stumbling block I saw was the low number of WS people known to us in Ireland. I decided to try out my idea!

I explained my idea to the member families via the newsletter. The feedback was positive so I went ahead and arranged a music weekend in Ballinasloe on 4th to 6th April 1997. It was a huge success. We ran music workshops on the Saturday morning, Saturday afternoon and Sunday morning. On Sunday afternoon we presented a "concert" that brought tears to the eyes of many present. I think I knew then that I had to try to use music to help the WS people in the future. The fact that the group that took part that weekend were not all musical "geniuses" told me that music could be used to help ALL WS people. That was what I wanted. There and then the seed that had been planted in my head about a music camp in Ireland began to germinate!

It was to take some time for the idea to come to full fruition! I put the idea to the WSAI committee and they seemed to think that it was a good one. They agreed to send myself and Karen to the camp in the USA in the summer of 1998 on a research mission. It turned out to be a very worthwhile trip! I learned so much from that first visit. It was to turn out to be the first of 6 trips to the camp for Karen. We were so impressed with the programme there and the way it was run that her father and I decided that we would bring her back again and again! Her final trip there was in 2003.

We came home from the camp in Belvoir Terrace, USA in summer 1998 full of enthusiasm for the idea of starting our own camp. But where to start? We had presented all the information we had collected to the committee and had received their blessing to proceed with the idea. I set about turning the idea into reality!

The first decision I made was that I was going to take my time with this project and do it right! I set summer 2000 (the millennium year) as my target for the first camp. The first task, I thought, was to find a venue. This took some time. Over the following months, my husband and I attended other camps and events with Karen in different locations just to check out the venues. Eventually I decided on the Share Holiday Village in County Fermanagh as the location for our camp. I felt it offered the best range of facilities and that it would be a secure environment for our WS people.

Having decided on the venue, I then started to try to organise the camp itself. I wanted it to emulate the camp in the USA but did not want it to be exactly like it. I would have to provide "helpers" for each of the WS campers and would also have to find all the teachers for the music programme as well as all the musical instruments! I felt we needed to be able to offer a family holiday to our members to encourage as many as possible to attend. So I came to a compromise. We would give the families three options—a music option, a music/activity option or an activity only option.

However, sometime into the preparations for the camp, Karen was selected as a member of the Irish Special Olympics team to participate in the Special Olympics European Games in Holland in June 2000! She was selected on the swimming team. That stopped me in my tracks! I realised how much of a drain on my time her preparations were going to be. We had to facilitate a training schedule locally as well as a training schedule with the team in Dublin once a month. We would also have to fundraise to cover her costs in Holland.

In hindsight, I am very glad that I made the decision that I did. I decided to postpone the first WSAI music camp until 2001 and commit my efforts to Karen for 2000.

So the first Music/Activity Camp happened in the Share Holiday Village in Fermanagh from 15th to 22nd July 2001. It was a wonderful event! All the hard work (and there was a lot of it!) was worth the effort when we watched a performance of "Joseph and his Amazing Technicolour Dreamcoat" at the end of the week! Everyone who was there gave so much to the week, all on a voluntary basis!

It was a very emotional culmination to the project for me

personally. I had nurtured the idea for so long and to finally see it fulfilled was a wonderful experience. I was told after the show that nobody on committee had really ever expected the idea to work!! Despite that, or maybe because of that, I would like to thank them all for the support and encouragement they gave me through the whole process.

I think the success of the project can be measured more fully now as we have just completed our 7th Annual Music/Activity Camp this year! I would like to acknowledge the financial support given to this project by many people. I would like to specially thank the National Lottery for the very substantial funding that they provided for the project. I do not think it would have been possible to have run the camp for the last 7 years without their financial help.

WSAI Story – 2nd Edition Update

IT IS NOW OCT 2012 and the members of the Williams Syndrome Association committee are busy putting the final touches to the plans for this year's AGM. This is a special year for the WSAI as it is the 25th anniversary of the founding of the association. Plans include speakers, music workshops and a disco, all to be followed by a gala celebratory dinner.

What a lot has happened in that 25 years! It is hard to believe all that has been achieved. As the incidence of WS is still given as 1:20,000, the number of WS people in Ireland is still relatively small. Over the years, we have probably had contact with somewhere between 80 and 100 families with a WS individual. I still think there are quite a few out there that remain undiagnosed, particularly in the older age groups. We continue to spread the word about WS as best we can. I am happy to say that, in recent years, we have made contact with a number of WS families in Northern Ireland. They are now beginning to join our association and take part in our activities. This is adding a whole new dimension to our organisation. Although the association was set up originally as an all-Ireland group, it is only in recent years that we have had interest from WS families in the North.

We are also finding that WS children are being diagnosed at a much younger age – some at only a few months of age. This, we feel, is very positive progress and we like to think that the WSAI has, in some way, helped to bring this situation about.

The WSAI is still a very active organisation with a very hard-working committee. Member families receive information on a regular basis via mailings, newsletters, etc. Annual activities organised for member families include weekend outings, day trips, informational seminars, AGM and, of course, the weeklong Music/Activity Camp in Fermanagh in the summer. The Music Camp has just completed its twelfth very successful year. It continues to attract WS campers from overseas as well as Ireland. Over the 12 years of its existence campers have attended from UK, Italy, The Netherlands, and Germany. It also continues to attract many volunteers from all parts of the world to work with our WS campers.

Many research projects have been supported by members of the WSAI over the years. Families are always very willing to take part and give of their time to answer questions, fill in questionnaires, take part in tests, etc. Some researchers have, in their turn, been very helpful to the WSAI by working as volunteers at the Music Camp, giving talks at our seminars, etc.

Finance and fundraising events continue to be at the top of the priority list for the WSAI committee. Many people have contributed to our fundraising efforts over the years. Many WS families and other wonderful friends have helped by making donations and by organising coffee mornings, race nights, musicals, balls, bag packing in supermarkets, taking part in sponsored walks, etc. etc., all to raise funds for WSAI.

The WSAI continues to have ongoing contact with the

other WS associations worldwide. It is a founding member of the European Federation of Williams Syndrome Associations (known as FEWS). This organisation has been in existence since July 1999 and is currently investigating the possibility of organising a European WS Convention in the near future. It continues also to organise an annual summer camp in one of its member countries. Irish WS people have participated in, and benefited from, some of these camps since they started in 2005.

Over its 25 years, I think the Williams Syndrome Association of Ireland has become a very important resource for the families of WS people. I think it has certainly achieved the aims for which it was founded and I hope it will continue to help and support many more WS families in the future. I think it has truly come of age!

My WSAI

WHAT HAS THE WILLIAMS SYNDROME Association of
Ireland given to me and my family?

HOPE when we despaired of what the future held for us
CONFIDENCE to face that future.
UNDERSTANDING of what it meant to be in our situation
INFORMATION when we needed it most and in a way that
was less painful to digest
ENCOURAGEMENT that things were not as bad as they
seemed and that life could still be good and very rewarding
FRIENDSHIP
COMPANIONSHIP
ACCEPTANCE...the list is endless.

What have we given to the WSAI in return?
Very little but I intend to change that, to give the little that
I can give which will be of any use i.e. support

Few of us realise just what the WSAI committee members
are doing behind the scenes. At best we tend to take this for
granted and, even worse, we do not take advantage of it. They

are there to help us when we need it, even if it is only for the tiniest snippet of information. They are always there in the background working away to ensure that we have recourse to them when we need them, asking only that we take advantage of them. I put my hand up now as one of the "offenders."

Last year I had my eyes opened to the wonderful work done by those who really do use the association and its gifts. I attended the 2005 AGM in the Lucan Spa Hotel and, afterwards, the very enjoyable show put on by the young WS people who had attended the annual music camp in Lisnaskea earlier that year.

The entertainment was mighty! You would not believe the talent and confidence shown by all on stage. There followed a presentation which gave a brief synopsis of what happens at the music camp, which is, everyone has a ball, pulls together, laughs a lot and goes a bit mad. Oh, and I almost forgot, they learn music! The reason I almost forgot that is not because it is a minor detail but that it is done in such a way that I don't think they even realise that they are learning but the end result definitely shows that they do.

Even those that are not particularly musical gain such fun and confidence from the experience that they get up on stage and give it as much as any professional entertainer. Looking around at the faces of parents watching their offspring on stage and realising, maybe even for the first time, that their child is a happy, whole, beautiful individual, capable of so much.

Believe me! Music is only one of the subjects learned at the camp. The others are confidence, friendship, positive image and self-respect.

The whole night was a very uplifting and moving experience. I wish that all WS families could have had this experience as I came away from there with renewed hope and happiness and determination that my son is a wonderful person, capable of so much and will reach his full potential.

I am going to take a more active role in the association from now on. That is my privilege and my gift, not to the association but to myself, as I know that I will gain more than I could ever possibly give. I also realise that not everyone can do very much.

Life is very busy especially for us with children with a disability. I am lucky that I have now come to a stage in my life when it has got a lot easier and doesn't seem such hard work. I am now ready to give something back (though I know it will be very little).

If, like me, you have never attended the music camp or even considered that it might be something that would benefit your WS son/daughter/sibling, I would encourage you to give it some thought. Anyone who has attended it will tell you what a wonderful, enjoyable and learning experience it is.

Karen's Story III

KAREN, HER FATHER AND I HEADED TO America in August 1998 to participate in the Music Camp run by the WS association over there. The trip had a dual purpose. I wanted to learn as much as I could about how the camp was run so I could recreate it in Ireland. I also wanted to find out if Karen really had any musical ability!

Karen had great difficulty settling into the camp environment. Campers were housed in wooden chalets along with their counsellors/helpers! We were in rooms in the main house—a beautiful old building! I think Karen had difficulty understanding why she could not be with us when we were so close by! She also had trouble with the American vocabulary e.g. a "dressing gown" suddenly became a "bathrobe," "toilet" was "rest room," etc. She just did not know what they were talking about half the time!

The biggest problem she had was with the food! Karen's main problem all her life had been food! Now she was expected to eat all manner of things she had never seen before. She did not eat anything! She existed on milk and tea and packets of chipsticks (courtesy of her mother!)

for the first three days. By Wednesday she was so hungry that she had to eat and she did—a little! However, this whole problem with the food meant that she really was not participating fully in the music programme. She went to all her classes and did what she was asked to do but she did not seem to be enjoying it very much.

On Wednesday we began to notice a little change. She seemed to be settling a little and began to enjoy the music. I began to look forward to Friday because on that day, we, the parents, were allowed to sit in on class and talk to the teachers. Karen (or I should say, I) had selected piano and guitar lessons as her two musical choices. Friday came and I spoke to the guitar teacher. Suffice it to say that Karen will never be a guitarist and she has never had a guitar lesson since! However, the piano teacher had amazing things to say about her ability and strongly advised me to get her piano lessons when we got home.

I was delighted! This was confirmation from people that should know that Karen had a keen ear for music and an ability to play piano. I vowed to arrange lessons for her as soon as we returned home. Up to that point, Karen had never had a music lesson. She played her keyboard at home many times every day but she had never been taught. This I would change now! This experience at the USA camp had shown me that she was now ready to take musical instruction. However, it would still need a very special teacher to work with her because she could not read music. I was advised by the teacher at camp that I needed someone that would teach her by "rote." I did not even know what that meant but I would find out and I would find her a teacher!

Karen performed on keyboard on the final night of camp and took part in the show. We were so proud of her!

We returned home and I found her teacher—a music teacher who was also a neighbour and friend and who was just starting a degree in Music Therapy at that time. She agreed to take Karen on as a pupil. It took them about three months to get used to one another and be able to work productively together. They have never looked back since and they are still together as teacher and pupil. I will be forever grateful to that teacher for taking Karen on as a pupil and teaching her so much. Karen now has a Bronze medal for piano and both Bronze and Silver medals for singing from the Royal Irish Academy of Music.

Karen's life now is a very happy one. She attends a day centre locally that is run by the Brothers of Charity Services. She is collected by bus each morning and delivered home each evening. She goes for respite breaks of 2 or 3 nights approximately once a month.

She is healthy enough. She still has checkups with the cardiologist and her paediatrician stills takes care of the other annual tests that she needs—mainly for kidney function. She tends to have slightly raised blood pressure all the time and, routinely, we have this checked over a 24 hour period. So far there has been no need for medication for this.

She still attends her piano and singing classes once a week during term time. She does not swim very much anymore. Sorry, I should say, she does not train for swimming any more! She just likes to go to the Special Olympics galas and win medals to show to her friends. I try to tell her that she needs to train in order to win the medals. Invariably she proves me wrong. She just turns up to the galas and wins medals anyway! How can I argue with that!

Karen is now 24 years of age. She has a very outgoing personality but does not relate to her peers very well. She prefers to spend her time on her own. She is a very loving friendly child who hates people to be upset.

Most WS individuals have obsessions and her obsessions are mainly with people. The love of her life is Pat Kenny of RTE. She has scrapbooks full of pictures of him and needs to go to see him at least once a year!

Karen's life is very full and, for her, content. Naturally, Paschal and I have all the worries that go with having a learning disabled child and we are doing our best to provide for her future. However, we are lucky! Karen has a brother who loves her deeply. I know that her best interests will always come first with him!

As parents we feel very lucky to have two Angels at Our Table.

Karen's Story
– 2nd Edition Update

KAREN IS NOW 29 YEARS OF AGE and very much looking
forward to being 30 next year! She expects a big party! She is
still happy and content with her life although I do now see some
tendency towards anxiety in her. She goes to the local Brother's
of Charity Adult Services five days a week and participates in a
varied programme comprised of social skills, computers, art &
craft work, gardening, etc.

She avails of fairly regular respite provided by the Brothers
of Charity Services as well. She gets roughly 3 respite breaks
over two months. These can be a 2 or 3 night break mid week
or a weekend break. While she enjoys going to respite, she is
always very happy to come home! I think she would opt to stay
at home all the time if given the choice!

She does not swim competitively any more but enjoys a
casual visit to the local leisure centre now and again. She is
still a very proficient swimmer and also enjoys using the gym
equipment, both in the leisure centre and in her day care centre.

She still attends her music lesson once a week during school
term and enjoys singing and playing the piano. However, I do
not hear nearly as much music being played in the house as I

Karen's Story
– 2ⁿᵈ Edition Update

used to! There was a time when she played her piano many times every day! She now spends more time listening to music on her CD player. She also spends a lot of time sitting on the sitting room floor playing on her iPad! She watches videos of the most amazing things on it – aeroplanes taking off, dogs barking, babies crying, washing machines spinning, wrestlers fighting, etc. She seems to be able to find anything she wants on it! She watches music videos ad infinitum! I regularly get questions like "What are the letters for ...." when she wants me to spell some word for her so she can Google it on the iPad!

Karen still spends lots of time on her own. She seems to enjoy being by herself and doing her own things like she always has. She loves to go outside (when the weather allows!) walking in the neighbourhood and "seeing her friends". When she has had a few words with "her friends", she returns home and gets on with her own stuff like watching TV, listening to music, playing with the iPad. These "friends" of hers are not her peers. They are the neighbours who have known her all her life, her doctor, the paediatrician who looked after her as a child, etc.

She still likes to have her life organised and to know what is happening each day. She likes to know what is being planned and gets upset if plans are changed at the last minute. She has learned to cope with change to some extent and does not get quite as upset by it as she used to. I suppose some of that comes with age and, of course, with life's experiences. She has had to cope with the loss of her father, Paschal, who passed away in Jan 2008 and the loss of her grandfather, Ted, who passed away last year. Her dad's death caused her to retreat back into herself a lot. She began to "mind" me as if she was afraid that I might leave her too! While she still has great difficulty talking about her dad, she does seem to have accepted that he is no longer with us and she is getting on with her day to day life.

I do not know what the future holds for her but, for now, she is happy and healthy and enjoys her life. I think that is all any of us can ask for!

Angel at my table

THE WORD "BLAME" has such negative connotations. Checking in the thesaurus as I write this, synonyms and associations include: culpability, guilt, impugn and to think badly of. None of these really apply here. However it remains the word I need, the word I use. I blame my sister for a lot.

My sister has Williams Syndrome. She is 18 now and is the most wonderful thing in my life. Coming up on 21 now, I am away at college and do not get to see her half as much as I would like. It's strange though. I'll be the first to admit, that even when I was at home I was more likely to be conning her into changing the TV channel than spending "quality" time with her. I was never great at doing things with her. Not "things" in the conventional thinking, I guess.

I rarely brought her outside to kick a ball with me. I don't think I ever did in fact. And, as I sit here and wonder why not, I know why not. She didn't want to. She had no interest in kicking a ball around. Trying to get her to kick a ball with me would upset her. I didn't want to upset her. All I ever wanted was for her to smile and laugh. Therefore, simple logic dictated that I should not try to get her to kick the ball around with me.

For as long as I can remember, my mother has been telling me that I need to encourage Karen to do "normal" things. I did. I encouraged her to do things that were normal to her. I wanted to see her smile, and do the things she enjoyed doing made her smile. Like anyone else, Karen went through phases in her life. She enjoyed certain things and then grew out of them while finding other things that made her happy. We went through a wrestling phase, where she loved watching wrestling and play wrestling with me. Now, when I'm at home, as I am saying goodnight to her on a Friday night, I find myself asking her if she will wake me up the following morning so we can watch wrestling. I don't know why I ask. She has no real interest in wrestling anymore. Yet, without fail, I still ask her every Friday night. Silly me!

I spent my summers, when I was old enough and responsible enough, minding Karen during the day while my parents were at work. From 9 to 4, Karen was my responsibility. We would watch TV, wrestle around, or maybe go to town so she could trawl through the magazines searching for pictures of Pat Kenny (probably the longest lasting of her phases has been her obsession with this TV personality!).

She would spend a good part of the day playing her keyboard. Music was always her first love. She is a musical genius. For a time, her music was just that—hers. I would be told in no uncertain terms that I had to leave whenever she wanted to play. That always hurt. It bothered me, and still does to this day, that her music is one thing I can't enjoy with her. She definitely got all the musical talent in our family. When she is playing her keyboard / piano, she is in her own world.

Her own world...I used to wait till she was in full flight and then sneak into the sitting room. I was never the most graceful, or stealthy of people, so getting in there unnoticed was a challenge to me. Many times she caught me and just stopped and looked at me. There was something in that look. It was as if she knew what I was doing and why I was doing it. I can't really explain it. Sometimes she told me again to leave, but other times her face almost seemed to pity me and decide to tolerate my presence. I would lie on the couch and listen.

My parents used to complain that we would spend too much time "lazing about the house" during those summer days. It wasn't lazing. It was our quality time. She did what she loved most, and I did what I love most—I watched her be happy.

I blame Karen for me. I blame her for me—the person I am. I am who I am because of Karen. Having an angel like Karen in my life has made me the person I am and the person I will become. From simple things like realising that people are different and knowing from an early age that everyone is special in their own way, to helping me realise who I am—Karen has given me so much.

I've had the pangs of resentment. They're no source of guilt for me. I don't believe I'd be human if I hadn't felt resentful of her at some stage. I never went through a stage of resentment so to speak but I have resented her in anger at various times, as I recall. The fact that I cannot remember any of these times distinctly, says a lot.

I've been embarrassed of her. I've found myself wishing the ground would swallow me. She is prone to little tantrums and I've found myself cringing when she's thrown one in public. Why me? Why does she have to be my sister?

One of the most wonderful and, indeed, most difficult things I have had to deal with concerning Karen is her increasing independence. It is great for her that she can do more things for herself and does not have to rely on others anymore. She used to rely on me a lot. It was a good feeling. I guess me feeling I've lost something as she has grown more independent is selfish. She doesn't need me like she used to. It's a good thing.

Karen has grown up a lot over the last few years in particular. She is doing things we never thought she would do. She developed a taste for salad. All those summers, I was cooking her sausages, beans and chips, as per orders. She is branching out and trying and enjoying new foods—something I thought she'd never really do.

I've missed a lot of it. I haven't been living at home for nearly 3 years now. She's changed a lot in those 3 years. It's hard for me to accept she's growing up and I'm missing it. Coming to college was tough for me. I never really considered not going to college, but it wasn't easy to actually pack up and do it.

I remember sitting around our kitchen table with my parents when I was about 12, and I had just finished primary school. I had done an entrance exam for a boarding school my father had attended. I had been offered a place and it was decision time. I was never going to go. I couldn't. I wouldn't have survived without her. I believe, back then, I was as dependent on her as she was on me. Even then I remember thinking, "I'll be away from her long enough when I go to college." I need(ed) her.

I am in Limerick, forging a life for myself. I have hopes and dreams. I want to achieve certain things in my life. Karen is always going to be my first priority. Her best interests are my primary interests. If that means making some tough decisions, so be it. Sin mar atá. If I believe it's in her best interest to be with me, she will be. If she will be better off somewhere else, so be it.

I must admit, the thought of Karen in full time care, away from me, does not appeal to me. I want to have her around. As it is, Karen does spend some time in respite care occasionally. She really seems to enjoy it. When my parents first broached the possibility with me, I was not immediately over-enthused. Selfishness and naivety again, I guess. It simply may not be practical, or in Karen's best interests, to be with me all the time. This is a realisation I have come to over a long period of time. We'll just have to wait and see how things work out.

Karen's a very lucky girl. She has the most wonderful parents anyone could hope for, and a brother who loves her dearly. Karen is our world. It hasn't always been easy and I hope it never will be. She knows how lucky she is. She is the smartest person I know. She knows how loved she is and that she will always be looked after.

This hasn't been easy for a 6"3,' 17 stone, tough guy bouncer to put on paper. While I am over-sensitive, not a lot of people know it. I hide it well from the people who need not know about it. The others, they know all too well.

Why me? Why does she have to be my sister? I guess I'm just blessed.

The Music Story

I HAVE ALREADY MADE MANY REFERENCES to the musical abilities of individuals with Williams Syndrome. Some WS people just love to listen to music, some love to have music around them all the time, some have a great ability to play a musical instrument and some have beautiful singing voices. Some can even compose their own music!

In July 2003, Brian attended the WSAI Music/Activity Camp in Lisnaskea, Co Fermanagh. This was Brian's second attendance at camp and, this time, he came prepared! He brought some of his own musical compositions with him! He had recorded these onto a tape and he presented me with a copy on the first evening at camp. I was very excited by this. It was the first time any of our Irish WS people had exhibited this ability. I passed the copy of the tape to our musical director that evening and she listened to it very intently. That was a Sunday evening!

By the following Tuesday night, some of the camp group, with the help of the musical director, had put lyrics to the newly composed music. The whole group listened enthralled that night to the first beautiful rendition of "Serenade; A Williams

Syndrome Anthem" and "Waves." That year at camp I promised Brian that his music would be properly recorded some day.

Over the following years at camp, other WS campers have composed pieces and put words to them as well. This year we have made a recording of some of this work and copies of the CD are available from the WSAI.

Serenade: A Williams Syndrome Anthem

Welcome to you all, to the Williams Family,
We're the best of good friends, you and me.
Come into our friendship, the Williams friendship tree
We're the best of good friends for all eternity.

And when you're low and feeling down and
You're in need; we're always there to help
Repeat All

New friends are good; it's hard to make new friends
So turn, shake hands with your neighbour
Spend some time and get to know your new friend
And you will find it does you good.
And when you're insecure and needing help
We're always there to help you

Welcome to you all, to the Williams Family,
We're the best of good friends, you and me.
Come into our friendship, the Williams friendship tree
We're the best of good friends for all eternity.

And when you're low and feeling down and
You're in need; we're always there to help

Respect your friends and it will be returned to you

Welcome to you all, to the Williams Family,
We're the best of good friends, you and me.
Ooh ooh

WAVES

Chorus   Today we should be thinking of our world
          Everyone for the sake of all mankind.
          Destruction, chaos, war and fear must end
          Or we'll not succeed in the saving of our world.

Verse One   Pollution is killing all our seas
             Cutting all our forests kills the trees
             So do your bit and save the world for you
             And you'll save it for your friends too.
             Chorus

Verse Two   Animals for experiment is cruel
             So is war for the sake of nuclear fuel
             So do your bit and save the world for you
             And you'll save it for your friends too.

Verse Three Accidental fire is killing all our wildlife
             Litter is ruining our streets
             So do your bit and save the world for you
             And you'll save it for your friends too.
             Chorus

             The environment should be important to us all
             Clean up your act, create a better place.
             So do your bit and save the world for you
             And you'll save it for your friends too.
             MAKE WAVES!

The contributions for this book have been penned by parents, in most cases by mothers, of individuals with Williams Syndrome. I include the following piece in this book of stories as a tribute to them.

"God Chooses Mom for Disabled Child"

Written by Erma Bombeck,
published in the Today Newspaper,
Sept 4th, 1993

MOST WOMEN BECOME MOTHERS by accident, some by choice, a few by social pressures and a couple by habit.

This year nearly 100,000 women will become mothers of handicapped children.

Did you ever wonder how mothers of handicapped children are chosen? Somehow I visualise God hovering over Earth selecting his instruments for propagation with great care and deliberation. As he observes, he instructs his angels to make notes in a giant ledger.

"Armstrong, Beth; son, patron saint, Matthew."

"Forrest, Marjorie; daughter, patron saint, Cecelia."

"Rudledge, Carrie; twins; patron saint... give her Gerard. He's used to profanity."

Finally, he passes a name to an angel and smiles, "Give her a handicapped child."

The angel is curious. "Why this one, God? She's so happy."

"Exactly," smiles God. "Could I give a handicapped child to a mother who does not know laughter? That would be cruel."

"But has she patience?" asks the angel.

"I don't want her to have too much patience or she will

drown in a sea of self pity and despair. Once the shock and resentment wears off, she'll handle it."

"I watched her today. She has that feeling of self and independence. She'll have to teach the child to live in her world and that's not going to be easy."

"But, Lord, I don't think she even believes in you."

God smiles.

"No matter. I can fix that. This one is perfect. She has just enough selfishness."

The angel gasps, "Selfishness? Is that a virtue?"

God nods. "If she can't separate herself from the child occasionally, she'll never survive. Yes, there is a woman I will bless with a child less than perfect. She doesn't realise it yet, but she is to be envied. She will never take for granted a 'spoken word.' She will never consider a 'step' ordinary.

When her child says 'Momma' for the first time, she will be present at a miracle and know it! When she describes a tree or a sunset to her blind child, she will see it as few people ever see my creations."

"I will permit her to see clearly the things I see—ignorance, cruelty, prejudice—and allow her to rise above them. She will never be alone. I will be at her side every minute of every day of her life because she is doing my work as surely as she is here by my side."

"And what about her patron saint?" asks the angel, his pen poised in mid-air.

God smiles.

"A mirror will suffice."